Animal Matters

CHARLOTTE REA

Animal Matters

DIARY OF AN INNER-CITY VET

CORONET

First published in Great Britain in 2019 by Coronet
An Imprint of Hodder & Stoughton
An Hachette UK company

This paperback edition published in 2020

1

A CIP catalogue record for this title is available from the British Library

Paperback ISBN 9781473694699
eBook ISBN 9781473694705

Typeset in Sabon MT by Hewer Text UK Ltd, Edinburgh
Printed and bound in Great Britain by Clays Ltd, Elcograf S.p.A.

Hodder & Stoughton policy is to use papers that are natural, renewable
and recyclable products and made from wood grown in sustainable
forests. The logging and manufacturing processes are expected to
conform to the environmental regulations of the country of origin.

Hodder & Stoughton Ltd
Carmelite House
50 Victoria Embankment
London EC4Y 0DZ

www.hodder.co.uk

TO JAMES

For giving me courage

AND TO MY PARENTS

For teaching me to cut the 't' out of can't

'Until one has loved an animal, a part of one's soul remains unawakened'

Anatole France

Prologue

Snowy was a beautiful white cat and he was my best friend. I was seventeen and he was fifteen when he was put to sleep. He had been in my life for longer than I could remember and as far as I was concerned he was as much a member of my family as I was. It was a miserable winter's night when it happened and the rain was unremitting. I hadn't seen Snowy all day. I heard the noise of the cat flap opening and went to investigate. He came in front feet first as he always did, but then I realised something wasn't quite right. He was dragging his back leg behind him and yowling a deep, throaty, anguished meow. I was horrified, and although it was nearly midnight, I woke my parents up to come and help.

My dad called the local vets, located the dusty cat box, which had not seen the light of day in over a decade, and we whisked him off to be checked out. The vet we saw was a gentle, caring and professional man in his thirties. He examined Snowy and decided to keep him there for pain relief and to do an X-ray and some blood tests. He listened to my concerns and calmed my fears, but made it clear all the same that things were not looking good. He didn't judge me when I sobbed my heart out on my father's shoulder and he was patient and understanding when we asked how much it would all cost. He didn't make us feel rushed, despite it being one o'clock in the morning and he didn't pressurise us into making a decision when we found out that Snowy's leg was fractured into several pieces and that his kidneys probably wouldn't survive the anaesthetic required to amputate it.

We took Snowy home for a few hours the next day to say goodbye. He sat on his favourite rug dosed up on painkillers and licked a Petits Filous out of the pot. One last treat before the end. I cuddled him and told him everything was going to be OK.

When I was a small child and he was a kitten, I would hold him with his head and front legs under my arm and his body and back legs hanging down like a ferret and we would walk around the garden for hours. He never wriggled or objected. I would put him in my doll's pram and wheel him about and he would sit there quite contentedly surveying the scene. He was the most tolerant feline I had ever met and he was my pal. He had seen me through many tantrums, school exams and my first relationship break-up when I had cried for days. He had slept on the end of either my bed or my sister's every night since we were all tiny. He had coped with us moving house and having builders in and out for years and tolerated my little brother coming along to wreck his peace even further. This was the first significant experience of loss I had faced in my life and certainly the first time I had actively had to make a decision on behalf of another being about the end of their life. I was heartbroken.

Later that day we took Snowy back to the vet for his euthanasia appointment. We saw the same vet we'd seen the night before. He must have been shattered after a night of broken sleep and a day consulting but he certainly didn't show it. He met us with a sympathetic smile and led us to a back room where he talked us through the procedure. When we were ready, he calmly and gently injected Snowy while we held him, tickled his chin and told him we loved him. The experience was surreal and emotionally exhausting but also peaceful and in some ways a relief after watching him suffer for the last twelve hours.

For many months afterwards I thought back to what had happened and I felt gratitude towards the vet for his manner and for allowing us to proceed at the pace we needed to, without either judgement or criticism. I never once felt like we were expected to keep Snowy alive when clearly the right thing to do was to let him go. But equally I didn't feel harassed into proceeding with his euthanasia before I was ready. The experience could have been so different if it had been handled by someone less compassionate. I felt inspired.

One year later I was sitting on a hammock in Guatemala with my oldest and best friend Kate, whom I have known all my life. Our chat turned from boys and travel plans to what we would be doing when we returned from Central America and how we felt about starting university.

'I feel very . . . meh,' I said.

'Why? Aren't you excited?' she asked.

'Yes, to be leaving home and starting something new, but not about the course I'm doing.'

I had applied to do psychology at Nottingham after being told by my teachers at school that I probably wouldn't get a place to do veterinary medicine. It's extremely competitive and they only take the best of the best, they had said. I didn't have what it took, or so I believed. I had watched as others applied and failed to get interviews, or got interviews and then received rejection letters, and I felt justified in my decision not to shoot for the stars.

But then I arrived in Central America. Our route had been planned at random and often changed last minute to add extra nights here and there. There was no online hostel booking back then; you just turned up with a backpack and a Lonely Planet guide and hoped for the best. But by some bizarre coincidence, along the entire route we travelled we were followed by two vets. They were older than us, women in their late twenties, and taking a career break.

After several weeks of eavesdropping on their conversations and jealously imagining what their lives and jobs were like, I finally summoned up the courage to speak to them. I asked them about their work and what university life had been like on the veterinary medicine course, and if they enjoyed their jobs. They told me that it was stressful and didn't pay well, and the on-call sucked. That they never finished on time. That the animals could bite, and the clients could be ungrateful and demanding, but

3

despite all this they couldn't think of anything else they would rather do.

Lying on the hammock it suddenly hit me. I had wanted to be a vet for a long time. Why hadn't I gone for it? I had been scared of failure, scared of rejection, and this fear had been exacerbated by the well-meaning but spirit-crushing advice from my teachers. I turned to Kate in a moment of rare gap-year clarity and said, 'I'm going to do it. I'm not going to Nottingham to do psychology. I'm going to become a vet.'

A year later I found myself surrounded by freshers in a pub in north London about to start veterinary school. I was thrilled to be given the opportunity to train as a vet and couldn't wait to get stuck into the course, but I was very nervous about fitting in. I had ended up taking an extra year out of education to get some experience working on farms and in stables, including a surreal two weeks spent living in a rusty caravan on a dairy farm with a tomcat called Romeo. I was a little bit older than most of the other undergraduates as a result, and felt slightly removed from freshers' life. The vet undergrads worked hard and partied hard, but having grown up in London and already done a fair bit of exploring, the party side of things didn't interest me as much. I needn't have worried though. I was lucky enough to meet a core group of like-minded people within my first couple of weeks who soon became my best pals. They remain so and have seen me through many of life's obstacles. Bizarrely and inexplicably, most of them are called Kate, or some variation of this. I seem to be a Kate/Katy/Katharine magnet. School aside, it was my first real taste of the necessity and importance of friendship in the face of a challenging working environment, something I would come to rely on increasingly as my career progressed.

On my first day at university I walked on to the campus to see a large banner outside one of the halls of residence rooms that read: BAN THE BAN ON FOX HUNTING. I was amazed that such a controversial topic would be approached in that way, and by people who would soon represent the voice of the veterinary profession. It was good for me in many ways to be surrounded by people from all over the UK, from the most urban of areas like me to the most rural and remote. I had spent my life thus far growing up alongside a fabulously eclectic mix of Londoners. The rural folk I had encountered on various camping and caravanning holidays in the New Forest during my childhood had been friendly and charming, but nonetheless very different to me and my urban reality. But now, in the middle of central London, it was time to shed the concepts of urban and rural and concentrate on a new and common goal: becoming vets.

The course itself was gruelling, fascinating, unrelenting and challenging in equal measure. Twenty per cent of my year either failed or quit within the first two years. It was certainly not for the faint-hearted. The vision of fifty beagle heads sitting on tables as we filed into the anatomy dissection class, not to mention the stench of old blood mixed with formalin, is etched into my mind for ever. Many of the most vivid memories I have from my university years involve the farm animal placements I attended. As a Londoner, I had had very little experience of working with farmers or cows until that point. One afternoon I spent several hours with my entire head and torso engulfed by the abdominal cavity of a cow that was hanging up by her forelegs in the post-mortem parlour, searching for the piece of metal fencing we suspected she had consumed and subsequently died from. We never found it, but if I hadn't known that a cow has four stomachs before that point, I certainly did after. I will also never forget the day I assisted in the castration of thirty five-month-old calves in a remote part of Yorkshire without any local anaesthesia. Those poor animals. It was not the first time I had witnessed animal cruelty and had not been able to speak up about it, and it wouldn't be the last. But I knew if I complained I might not be signed off for my farm animal placement, a compulsory part of my course. And so I watched and tried to seem interested and eager rather than disappointed and dismayed as the animals kicked out in pain.

At the end of the session, the vets and farmers started to collect the testicles in long rectal gloves. At first I assumed they were just rounding them up to put them in the clinical waste bin, until one of the farmers turned and offered me a glove.

'They taste delicious fried up with a bit of butter and flour,' he said with a wink.

I took them apprehensively as I couldn't muster the gumption to tell him that I was slightly disgusted by the concept. Or that I was vegetarian, which would have been as frowned upon in that environment as an atheist in a Catholic church. *Perhaps this is just the way it's done in rural England*, I thought.

Later that evening I collected the sweaty rectal glove from the boot of my car and offered my harvest to my friend Kate's parents whom I was staying with. They looked dubiously at the glove and Kate's dad smiled politely and her mum giggled nervously. Half an hour later we were tucking into a vegetable lasagne and the glove containing all six testicles was sitting firmly in the bin. For the record, rural or urban, I have since learned that the law states that all castrations of calves over the age of two months must be done using anaesthesia. I'm still waiting for the law on eating testicles to come into place.

The clinical years at vet school were a blur of long arduous night shifts, lectures, presentations, seeing practice at first-opinion veterinary practices during 'holidays', and revising for the all-important finals in every spare moment. This, intermingled with abundant cups of tea at each other's houses and boozy nights celebrating birthdays and end of rotation blocks. It was exciting to finally have the opportunity to work 'hands on' with the animals after years of burying my head in books. There was a buzz about it, despite the exhaustion. But there was also a feeling of exhilaration mixed with terror as the end approached, knowing that very soon the buck would stop with me. No more cushioning or asking teachers for advice about every case. In the final few months before graduation I began to feel like an impostor, entirely unqualified to write those three little letters on any form asking for my profession. Vet. How could I do this job justice?

During some student placements throughout my clinical years at university it had been a struggle to even work out which flea or worming treatment I should be offering clients with the plethora of different products currently available. I would listen to vets consulting who had only a few years of clinical experience and watch in awe as they handled difficult clients or complex medical cases. I couldn't imagine ever reaching a point where I would be that competent or efficient. I had performed a handful of spays and castrations by this point, and many basic consultations and vaccinations, but always with my clinical rotation group and a veterinary clinician by my side, or at least on the other side of the door. But soon I would be expected to know the answers without help. To operate on animals and recognise what diseases they were suffering from. To fix them. To euthanise them. Owners would lay their trust in my hands, and I couldn't disappoint. And then, without any further opportunity to dissect the moment, it suddenly happened. Five years of intensive training had come to an end and I was a vet.

During my training I had decided pretty early on that I wanted to become a small animal vet. My friend Mark, who is not a vet, once asked me how small an animal had to be to be considered a 'small animal'. He assumed a 'small animal vet' means you only treat teeny, tiny creatures like mice. This made me laugh. For the sake of clarity, it generally means dogs and cats (and rabbits, hamsters, ferrets and other small furry creatures) as opposed to farm animals or horses. I had a great deal of respect for the beauty and strength of large animals, and had greatly enjoyed my farm animal rotations despite the overwhelming feeling that my arm simply wasn't long enough to feel all the important structures inside a cow. It sure is warm inside there on a winter's day though.

But my innate affinity was with dogs and cats. I understood them. I felt natural in their presence having grown up around them as a child in a way that I didn't feel with horses or cows.

Some time before graduation I had decided that I wanted to work in the charity sector. I had wandered around the careers tables at veterinary shows during my final year at university showing vague interest in the private practice stands, both corporate and independent, but I knew deep down that my dream job was to work for an animal charity in London.

There is no equivalent to the NHS in the vet world. Animal charities are relatively few in number and are spread thinly, mainly around large cities such as London and Manchester and on the south coast. We are extremely lucky to have them at all. Most other countries around the globe have animal welfare charities but very few offer veterinary services for free or low-cost treatment. Every year the Pet Food Manufacturers' Association (PFMA) commissions a 'Pet Population' report which looks in detail at pet ownership trends. In 2018, approximately 12 million (45%) of UK households were reported to have pets. This included nine million dogs and eight million cats, leaving many clients on low incomes, or who had hit hard times, struggling to pay their vet bills. Pet ownership is extremely rewarding, but can also be disconcertingly costly. This is highlighted by the fact that, according to the Association of British Insurers (ABI), pet insurance companies settled a million claims, paying out £775 million in 2017 for the first time in the industry's history. Pet owners are relying increasingly on insurance because many people simply can't afford to pay for the range of treatments available to restore their beloved pet's health. But what happens to the percentage of society who can't even afford the insurance costs? There is speculation that people should not own pets if they are unable to afford their veterinary care, but in my experience these are often the members of society who need their companionship the most.

I felt immediately connected to all the staff members I met at the veterinary charities where I'd spent time as an undergraduate.

I'd been blown away by the facilities and extremely high quality of care I had come across, and amazed by the low-cost or donation-based treatment options offered to pets belonging to some of the least fortunate members of society. People who were illiterate, had suffered terrible abuse or whose disabilities meant they were housebound, but whose pets made the difference between enduring a miserable lonely existence and living a life filled with love and meaning.

One charity stood out to me in particular, and I dreamed of working for them, of being a part of it all. For the sake of discretion I will refer to this organisation as the Pet Welfare Hospital (PWH). At over 120 years old, and caring for over 40,000 pets each year, I found it astounding that PWH received no government funding whatsoever and relied entirely on legacies and donations to help pay for the cost of rehoming unwanted animals, providing veterinary services and promoting animal welfare. Although there is generally a shortage of vets in the UK (an issue which will only be made worse by Brexit, but that's another story), it is still extremely difficult to get a job as a newly qualified vet in a busy inner-city London animal charity hospital. Life is fast-paced, and usually requires a level of skill not yet acquired by a fresh-faced, poorly experienced vet on day one out of university. So I began my post-university veterinary life as a locum. This essentially meant temporarily filling the role of a permanent member of staff who was unavailable for any reason. Many vets chose to locum permanently or as a stopgap between jobs, moving around different practices as needed to give them more freedom and better pay. Unfortunately, I'm not that cool and I am a stickler for routine and job security. I knew as soon as I started that I wanted to find something more permanent and I could not ignore this niggling desire to move into the charity orb. So when, after several months of working as a locum in private practices and feeling slightly lost, I was offered a job at one of PWH's main hospitals, I was absolutely thrilled. There was no doubt in my mind that I would take it.

*

To say that my first few years in clinical practice were a huge learning curve would be a vast understatement. There is no amount of training that can prepare you for the emotional and physical energy required to work regular twenty-six-hour shifts, deal with clients who often have serious mental health problems, work tirelessly to achieve the best standards of care you can for the highest number of pets possible in the face of relentless pressure from clients, managers and, more disconcertingly, from yourself. Within two years I was unrecognisable from the new graduate who had entered the building on day one.

I had what would be considered by many to be a privileged upbringing. Two parents who had made me feel loved and cherished, two siblings with whom I got on very well, a safe roof over my head and the support needed to become whatever I wanted to be. I had been exposed to very little in the way of heartache, other than losing my beloved Snowy. I was therefore underprepared for the degree to which I would be expected to act as a counsellor to my clients as well as a doctor to their pets.

I received daily verbal abuse like I had never been exposed to before and experienced tiredness levels that were far worse than the exhaustion I had felt as a student. I learned how to perform euthanasias sometimes under the worst or saddest of circumstances, and how to muster immediate enthusiasm for the puppy vaccination that followed straight after. I learned to hide emotion when I was unable to cure terminally ill patients belonging to vulnerable clients whose hearts were breaking because of their loss, and developed a deep sense of guilt associated with these sad cases that lingered for some days and followed me home. But I was also in love with the job. I lived and breathed it, staying late to write up cases and scrub in on new surgeries, socialising in the evenings in the pub opposite the hospital with my work colleagues as we dissected the day's events. I was amazed by how trusting, friendly and resilient many of my clients were. Putting aside the hideousness of the rush-hour commute, I actively looked forward to going to work each day and chatting to new people about their lives, observing them from a unique viewpoint as they unfolded in front of me. But most of all I felt privileged to be a part of the special and often profound bond people have with their pets.

Several years into the job, I was having dinner with my family and discussing some of the more poignant and funny cases I had come across in recent weeks (all personal details omitted of course). My father, a forensic psychiatrist with an abundance of his own fascinating clinical stories, suggested I start writing a diary of my cases. I laughed at the time and dismissed it, but later that week I found myself purchasing a new writing book. I had always written diaries as a young girl and when I was travelling as a teenager. I thought it might be fun and therapeutic to start noting down some of my cases, and once I started I found I couldn't stop. I would arrive home following a night shift, full of adrenaline and with an overstimulated and overburdened brain that made sleep impossible, and I would scribble down my thoughts until my mind was clear. As I wrote I realised how little people knew about the work vets actually do, and how much of a toll it can take on our lives, however magical it can also be. I recently rediscovered my diary entries and found myself crying tears of joy and sadness as I reminisced about the animals and people who had touched my life during that time. I decided it was time to share them to provide a glimpse to the outside world of this crazy whirlwind profession we vets live, but also to stand up for a profession that isn't always spoken about kindly, and which I fought hard and feel privileged to be a part of. All diary entries are based on real-life cases but patient, client and colleagues' names and details have been altered where necessary to maintain confidentiality. There will be some explanations of medical terms along the way and the more complex cases and issues will be contextualised where necessary. But the rest are just the facts and feelings of a city vet.

Part One

AUTUMN

Just finished a shift consulting alongside a new veterinary graduate. She was volunteering to gain some experience prior to getting her first job. Volunteering as a newly qualified vet is quite a common scenario around the London area, unless you're happy to take a job in Northumberland as a mixed small and farm animal vet working for peanuts and on-call every other weekend. She was perfectly capable and had the right balance between confidence and knowing when to ask for help. Despite her aptitude it reminded me quite how steep the learning curve is for new veterinary graduates and how much you are thrown in at the deep end. All the way home on the tube I was laughing and cringing to myself reminiscing about my early days in my first job. My very first consultation was Bert the budgie who had been brought in with a sore wing. Most vets reading this will now feel a pang of sympathy for me. I'm pretty sure avians were allotted only one day of lectures during my five years of undergraduate training. I'm also pretty sure I bunked these lectures as I was on a second date with James, my then boyfriend, and now long-suffering husband. And so began a frantic google search to find all possible causes of budgie wing issues.

Bert was actually pretty cute for a caged pet bird and I cooed over him for several moments, giving him the standard 'aren't you a lovely little fella, look at your sweet little face' etc. Every vet knows that whatever the animal looks like, you must always compliment it, even if it resembles Grumpy Cat with a hangover. I stood back observing him and assessing his cage husbandry before reaching in to have a look at him. He had a very tiny wound on one wing, which I suspected he had caught in the cage bars. Unfortunately, Bert had speed as well as looks on his side, despite his gammy wing, and he didn't appreciate my big fingers manhandling his slight 40g frame. He swiftly bit my hand and flew past me into the room, at the very moment my colleague was assessing a three-legged cat in the adjoining consultation room. And so began 'the chase'. Like a less funny version of Tweetie Pie and the Puddy-Tat, with the addition of the idiot vet, I began frantically stumbling around trying to grab the budgie as my colleague tried to grab the cat, who was stealthily hunting the blissfully unaware budgie, all running around a rather disgruntled-looking owner.

Eventually, after what was probably only a few seconds but felt like an eternity, the three-legged cat, who was struggling to jump on to the table following his recent change in balance, was pinned down by his owner, while Bert proudly settled himself on the door-frame hinge. Like a ninja, I sprang to the door and locked it, as images of the receptionist opening the door and creating a flat Stanley version of Bert ran through my mind. As I did so, the words of my university professor sprung to mind – 'Even if you feel things are spiralling wildly out of your control, always act with poise and confidence.' And with that little boost I casually threw a towel over Bert, clambered on to the chair and grabbed him from the door frame. I jumped down, smiled, popped him back in his cage and said, 'Just checking he can still fly well, and he can. It's a small wound and should heal on its own. Let's monitor for now and reassess in a few days.' And sure enough, a few days later at the recheck appointment, Bert's wing was right as rain.

Moral of the story: if you pick a budgie as your first ever consultation, make sure the cat in the adjoining room only has three legs.

4 SEPTEMBER 2014

All the vets decided yesterday that we would start a new trend of leaving work on time. We made a pact that we would leave at 5pm. This is our average contracted end of shift time which sounds gloriously civilised, in theory. In practice it is extremely rare for us to leave on time.

I was on a late shift today, which meant working until 9 p.m. Immediate fail! The standard practice is for the vet on the late shift to take over the outstanding procedures that need finishing and see any emergencies coming in, in addition to looking after the inpatients. We can have up to 30 sick animals staying in the hospital at any one time. At 5pm I finished consulting and came up to the 3rd floor for case handover – this is where all the action takes place. I walked into the ultrasound room to find my veterinary colleague, Lola, draining fluid from a dog's chest. This didn't look good. After a brief chat about the case, I went to check what else was going on. I walked into minors to find another vet colleague, Lucy, resuscitating an elderly cat that had taken a bad turn under anaesthetic. Minors is our short term for 'minor operations' and is the place where lump removals, dentals, cat castrations, wound dressings, X-rays, etc. take place. Basically anything that isn't major surgery. Majors, as you can probably guess, stands for 'major operations' where all the sterile surgeries take place, from routine procedures like spays and dog castrations, to orthopaedics and gastro-intestinal surgeries.

I assisted Lucy for several minutes until the situation was under control and then went through to radiography to find a nurse monitoring an anaesthetised cat that had been in a road traffic accident (RTA) and was having X-rays for suspected chest and pelvic trauma. Another very sick patient. Oh God. I went through into majors to discover that Sarah, another vet and good friend, had just gone into theatre with a German Shepherd with a bleeding splenic tumour that needed emergency surgical intervention.

Bugger.

Now came the decision of whom to relieve. If I went into theatre I would be in there for over an hour and I knew there were also at least two inpatients that needed assessing, plus two emergencies booked in and on their way down to the hospital. I could take over from Lucy but she was heavily involved with the case and would most likely want to follow through and speak to the owner herself. I dashed into the X-ray suite and checked the RTA cat and assessed his X-rays. Fractured pelvis and bruised lungs. Ouch. He would need stabilisation overnight and most likely require surgery tomorrow. I gave the nurse the OK to wake him from his anaesthetic and rushed back to ultrasound. My colleague handed me a sample of chest fluid to take to the lab for immediate interpretation. We assessed the heart scan together and discussed the case further. She wanted to continue with the procedure, which gave me a chance to assess the fluid under the microscope, check the inpatients, and see the new emergencies coming in. There were now four booked in and the first one – a vomiting dog – had already arrived.

Two hours later, 7pm, and all three of my veterinary colleagues were still working, writing up cases and calling owners. It occurred to me that without their help, my shift would have spiralled utterly out of control. It also occurred to me that this is not a one-off for us. This is pretty standard vet life. Sometimes I wonder what I would do without them, this crazy dysfunctional veterinary family of mine. I know they would never abandon me when I needed them, and I would do the same for each of them in a heartbeat. Although it's obviously a big part of it, working far beyond the end of our contractual shift times is not solely for the love of and dedication to the animals, and it's certainly not for career advancement and learning purposes. Not at that time of night after a ten-hour working day, anyway. It's for each other.

Needless to say, after a hopeless attempt at finishing on time, we have decided to abandon 'mission: finish on time' in favour of the alternative and more achievable 'mission: let's go to the pub'.

8 SEPTEMBER 2014

Today's first six appointments:

1. anal glands
2. anal glands and hair loss

3. sticking out anus
4. pussy wound (This one created much amusement among the nurses. The reception team is generally responsible for booking animals' appointments and their choice of words can lead to great hilarity behind the scenes.)
5. anal glands
6. penis stuck out

Whoever said this was a glamorous job?

10 SEPTEMBER 2014

I have just attended a professional development course on echo-cardiography (scanning hearts). To keep up to date and ensure we aren't practising archaic medicine, all vets have to complete 105 hours of courses, lectures and private study in any three-year period. This particular course involved eight hours of feeling overwhelmingly inadequate interspersed with breaks for bad coffee and soggy sandwiches. And, of course, paying £800 for the privilege. During one of these breaks, one of the other vets on the course, a young man in his mid-late thirties called Adam, started chatting to me about his veterinary work. Adam owns a large private practice in the Midlands. He asked me where I worked, and I told him, at which point he leaned in with a very serious expression on his face and asked me, 'What's that bright light?'

In my naivety I looked around me to find the bright light, only to be met with the dull headache-inducing glare of the university ceiling lights.

'What light?' I asked, confused.

'That light,' he continued, pointing at my head. 'Oh,' he continued, 'it must be the halo shining off your head.'

At this stage I realised he was attempting at best some ice-breaking banter and at worst a spot of cruel sarcasm related to the fact that I work for an animal charity. I found it neither remotely funny nor endearing but managed to force a small fake laugh.

He then dealt the major blow, 'Do you think you will be able to get a job at a normal vets after working to lower standards for so long at a charity?'

Now, I have come to expect this kind of comment from members of the public who perhaps aren't aware that us vets all go to the same universities; there are no 'charity vet universities' where we are taught to practise inferior medicine. Countless times, I have been on the receiving end of comments from clients such as, 'I used to have a job, and take my pets to a real vet, you know, a proper vet, but we've fallen on hard times so have to make do with you for now.' I can understand to some extent why there would be some confusion, as charities do have a low budget and we are restricted in terms of what we are able to do based on providing the highest quality of care to the greatest number of pets we can help. But what a lot of people, and clearly this particular vet, don't realise is that investigations in private practice are perhaps even more restricted, based on client budget, and a great deal of the more complex cases are referred. We are particularly lucky where I work to have five floors, two theatres, seven consulting rooms, two floors of kennels with separate dog and cat wards, an isolation unit, dozens of experienced nurses and 24-hour inpatient care. The quality of our work is by no means substandard. So I can forgive 'charity vet snobbery' from my clients, but I can't forgive it from a fellow vet. The veterinary community is small and we have to look out for one another. Needless to say, I avoided Adam for the rest of the day.

11 SEPTEMBER 2014

Today I saw Mr Koleki with his eight-year-old unneutered Staffie Freddy. 'Staffies' are our nickname for one of the most common breeds we see at PWH, the Staffordshire Bull Terrier. These dogs have been overbred to a terrifying degree in cities in the UK and are often used as fighting dogs. They have been painted by many as aggressive and unpredictable and given the title of 'status dogs', associated with gang culture. In my experience this is far from the truth and these dogs are usually affectionate and loving when brought up in the right environment. Sadly, Staffies in the UK are often abandoned by their owners. In 2013 more than a third of the dogs in the Battersea Dogs and Cats Home were Staffies, many of which had to be euthanised due to an inability to find suitable homes for them. Since then, they have continued to flood UK animal shelters and even more distressingly, the RSPCA has confirmed that 80% of its cruelty-to-animals prosecution cases involve Staffies.

Me: We recommend castrating Freddy, Mr Koleki. Unfortunately, as a charity, we can't support breeding. Freddy also has an inherited hip condition and could pass that on to his puppies. Plus, he is getting a bit older now, and we worry about prostate problems and testicular cancer which would be prevented by castrating him.

Mr Koleki: No way am I getting his balls chopped off. I wouldn't do it to myself, so why would I do it to him? [Mr Koleki cups his own anatomy with his hand, crosses his legs and grimaces as if in pain at the thought.]

Me: Mr Koleki, I can understand your point of view, but you are not a dog. You are a human. Freddy is living the lifestyle of a domesticated dog, and is crippled by arthritis caused by his hip dysplasia. At the very least, you shouldn't be using him for breeding.

Mr Koleki: So you're saying I should prevent him getting his leg over just because you say so? With all due respect, love, you're a woman. You don't understand about the needs of men. You claim to love animals and yet here you are trying to torture them!

Me: Mr Koleki, rehoming centres across the country are inundated with abandoned bull breeds, particularly Staffies like Freddy, many of whom we are struggling to find homes for. My concern is about the health and well-being of animals, which

includes Freddy and his future offspring. He wouldn't be missing out on anything if he were neutered at this late stage in his
life. In fact, he may end up living a longer and healthier life.

Mr Koleki: Let's just agree to disagree on this one, shall we? But
I'm telling you now, no one is going near my dog's balls unless
it's to make him happy! [Mr Koleki winks at me and wanders
off to collect more painkillers for Freddy's hips.]

Me: [Sighs.]

12 SEPTEMBER 2014

Today I started the day feeling positive. I was going to have a good
day. First appointment – 'Gentle Puss Puss'. The owner, Mr Patel,
was insistent on using his cat's full name throughout the consultation. Needless to say, Gentle Puss Puss had spent the first few
years of her life as a hungry and angry stray, otherwise known as
'hangry Puss Puss'. Being hangry and probably cold and unloved
had left Gentle Puss Puss with a rather understandably bad attitude by the time Mr Patel had adopted her two years ago.
Nonetheless, he had gallantly battled on and developed a rapport
with Gentle Puss Puss and now they lived together side by side,
Mr Patel accepting of the occasional unprovoked biting attack
and Gentle Puss Puss enjoying a new life of warmth, good food
and security. Thus bringing us to today. Mr Patel had woken up to
discover that Gentle Puss Puss was, alas, limping on her back leg.

Sure enough, she arrived holding her right back leg up
completely, at an odd angle, and I immediately suspected a fracture. Approximately ten seconds into the examination, I established that Gentle Puss Puss was indeed rather intolerant of being
handled. A savage attack followed on both myself and Mr Patel,
who continued to lavish Gentle Puss Puss with love and kisses,
which led to a swipe so close to his eyeball I was sure a trip to
A&E would need to follow. Stage two and Sophie, one of the
experienced veterinary nurses who is far better at handling savage
beasts than I am, came to assist and deemed it time to bring out

the big guns, aka the gauntlets. If you ever take your cat to the vet and they have to bring out the gauntlets, you know they mean business. You also know your cat is a bit of an arse. Unfortunately, our 'big guns' were also met with failure. Stage three and it was time to reach for the only weapon a vet has that places them in a position of superiority over any aggressive animal: drugs. Ah, wonderful, fast-acting, muscle-relaxing, mind-numbing sedatives. Several moments later Gentle Puss Puss was away with the fairies and ready for her X-ray.

Me: one; 'previously-hangry-now-called-gentle-but-actually-savage Puss Puss': nil.

16 SEPTEMBER 2014

Feeling pretty chuffed. Emma, one of the very experienced, very funny but no-nonsense nurses I've been working with for a long time, has finally started to call me by my name today. Hurrah! After years of being referred to as 'veterinary' ('Pass me that catheter, Veterinary', 'Your inappetent cat has started to eat, Veterinary'), today it was, 'Your constipated dog has just done a massive dump, Charlotte.' I feel like I have been given a promotion! I never quite managed to reach the first name status at university – I was 'student' until the day I left. And though I had come to see being called 'veterinary' by Emma as a term of endearment, I still feel like I have finally been accepted into some sort of special first name club. It's the little things in life . . .

19 SEPTEMBER 2014

I'm shattered today after being up half the night looking after my cat Bea, who decided to vomit every hour from midnight onwards all over the flat. She looked pretty rough this morning as I left for work and I knew I would worry about her all day. It's funny how having your own pet changes you as a vet. I adopted Bea in 2011 when she came into the hospital as a skinny five-month-old stray with a severely fractured leg, referred from another veterinary practice who didn't have the funds to treat her. I walked into kennels one Saturday morning on-call and saw her dragging herself across the table, her fractured leg flailing behind her. She was desperately trying to reach the tin of tuna one of the nurses had left out. I tickled her chin and she purred like a motorcycle and then proceeded to bite my hand in a fit of over-stimulation. For anyone who is not familiar with cats, this is the classic behaviour felines exhibit in response to too much petting. They become easily overwhelmed by seemingly inconsequential or previously pleasurable actions. They are complex creatures, which is partly why I love them.

We operated on Bea's leg that week but there was still a chance that it might need amputating so I took her home 'temporarily' to foster her while it healed. James told me on the phone that evening that he wasn't a cat person, and that at worst he would tolerate her and at best he would be indifferent to her. He walked through the door from work twenty minutes later and Bea climbed up on to his chest, nuzzled down and fell asleep. Sold. From that moment on they have been best friends and have even been known to eat their dinner from the same plate (not behaviour I would recommend as a veterinary professional, obviously).

She resided in a large cat kennel half the size of my postage-stamp living room for several weeks after she first arrived, during which time she chewed the bars of the cage door, continuously trying to escape. One evening she also managed to get her head around the edges of her plastic Elizabethan collar, affectionately known as the 'cone of shame', and managed to chew her stitches out. I thought I had become pretty hardened, that I would be a sensible and pragmatic cat owner. But from the moment this little ball of fluff landed on my doorstep my brittle exterior crumbled. I spent many nights lying awake worrying about the infection that had developed around the pins in her leg. What if her leg suddenly fell off overnight? I took her into work three times in one week seeking reassurance from my tolerant and understanding colleagues. What if she managed to escape the kennel while I was at work and damage the fracture site of one of her other legs? She could end up legless! I even stayed up one night until 2 a.m. sewing some material I found on to the edge of my old Brownie sash to create a new supersized soft E-collar for her. She thanked me by getting it caught in the cage door and then in a fit of feline anger ripping it to shreds the next day. Bye bye, Brownie sash, complete with six badges.

So there I was, a sane and rational vet and at the same time an utterly neurotic pet owner. I had a sudden newfound patience for owners who complained that they were not able to cage rest their animals because they were 'going crazy' in the cage. I no longer chastised owners of pets who had chewed out their sutures, 'these things happen'. I could completely identify with the panic in an owner's eyes when they brought their pet in worrying their fracture or other wound wasn't healing properly. I had become 'that type of owner'. The funny thing is that most vets are like this with their own pets. We find objectivity almost impossible and are overly anxious and sentimental about them in ways we rarely are about our patients. I can maintain calm in the face of a Great Dane having a seizure or an animal having a tumour the size of a melon removed from its abdomen, but when Bea gets a splinter in her toe I am horrified. But I suppose that's the point – our pets are our family members and our patients are just that – our patients. We have to keep it objective or we wouldn't be able to bear the heartache of it.

I returned home to a hungry, non-vomiting and brighter-looking moggie tonight. She raised a ginger eyebrow as I unpacked my enormous collection of work goodies, which included a bag of intravenous fluids complete with needles and syringes, some opioid-based painkillers, dehydration electrolyte sachets, anti-vomiting drugs, antacids and some tins of bland prescription cat food. Turns out I didn't need any of it as she scoffed a plate of her usual food then pottered out to the garden to hiss at the neighbour's dog. Crisis over.

22 SEPTEMBER 2014

Me: I noticed you didn't attend the recheck appointment we booked for Chico last week.

Owner: No, sorry, I couldn't make it.

Me: Any particular reason why? It's important we make sure we redress Chico's fractured leg regularly.

Owner: Yeah, sorry, I was on the *Jeremy Kyle Show* that day.

Me: . . . !

Best excuse for a missed appointment ever?

25 SEPTEMBER 2014

I performed my first solo airway surgery yesterday, or BOAS surgery as it is called by vets, on a French Bulldog called, imaginatively, 'Frenchie'. Brachycephalic Obstructive Airway Syndrome' (BOAS) refers to a group of conditions resulting from the body conformation of brachycephalic dogs (dogs with short noses), including breeds such as French and English Bulldogs, Pugs and Pekingese. I finished the surgery feeling utterly depressed. Frenchie is a six-year-old male dog who, like many brachycephalics, can't really breathe. He has struggled for years to walk more than a few metres without his tongue and mucous membranes (gums) turning slightly blue and in the summer his owner can barely take him out.

In veterinary medicine, as in human medicine, we often assess the colour of an animal's mucous membranes to provide information on their oxygenation. If a dog or cat's gums are pink, their body is likely to be reasonably well oxygenated. White, grey or blue (cyanotic) mucous membranes are alarming and tell us that an animal is struggling to pump enough oxygenated blood around their body to their cells. Sadly, many brachycephalic dogs spend a significant proportion of their lives bordering on cyanosis and Frenchie was one of these cases.

Frenchie spends the hot months of the year sprawled out in

front of a fan in the shade of the house, compensating for his obstructed airway by panting and pulling in air in great gasping snorts. He also has allergic skin disease, chronic ear disease – the latter a consequence of the former – dental disease and a creaky spinal disc that flares up from time to time. But, frankly, these are the least of his troubles.

When he arrived I could hear him coming a mile off. He had to be placed immediately into an oxygen supplemented kennel because the stress and excitement of sitting in a waiting room full of other dogs had made his breathing deteriorate. I discussed the risks of surgery with his owner, Miss Edmondson, and we went through the procedure. I explained that I would be widening his nostrils and trimming his overly long soft palate and that the surgery would hopefully improve his breathing, but that sadly nothing could completely reverse the effect that his severely abnormal facial conformation and skull anatomy would have on his long-term quality of life. Best-case scenario, we would improve his ability to run around and live like a normal dog. Worst-case scenario, he would continue to struggle to breathe every day for the rest of his life, or even die suddenly from his condition.

Once he was up in theatre I induced anaesthesia and as I went to place the tube to secure his airway, I realised that there was so much excessive tissue at the back of his throat that only a cat-sized tube, less than half the diameter of the usual tube used for a dog his size with a normal nose, would fit. I managed to place it, by-passing all the flesh at the back of his throat, and immediately started to supplement oxygen. Thankfully, he quickly went from a greyish colour to a lovely healthy pink. The nurse and I exchanged a look of relief and I realised we had both been holding our breath. Being under general anaesthesia was probably providing Frenchie's cells with the best oxygen supply they had ever had.

It is fiddly trying to operate at the back of a dark hole, but I had performed several like this previously with colleagues assisting and knew what to expect. The surgery went smoothly and I was pleased with the end result. Recovery is always a nerve-wracking part of the procedure as once the tube supplementing oxygen has come out, you are relying once again on a dog with a severely abnormal and now slightly swollen post-operative throat and nose anatomy to draw a normal volume of air down into their lungs. With a bit of a cough and splutter Frenchie started to breathe on his own and once again our relief was palpable. We carried him from theatre down to the dog kennels and placed him back into an oxygen cage to continue his recovery. I stood in front of his kennel for a long time watching him while the nurses continued to hustle and bustle around me, giving medication to other inpatients, taking the next patient up to theatre, monitoring a sick seizuring patient in the kennel next door. I felt suspended in time. How could we, as a society so concerned with animal welfare, let this happen?

Now don't get me wrong, I think Frenchies are pretty sweet looking. And Pugs come to that. They are often cutie pies with lovely natured cuddly personalities. I have fallen in love with many of them along the way and there are a number of 'healthy' ones out there who only have mild respiratory disease and have a good quality of life. Many of the flat-faced breeds are well established after all, and brachycephalic dog skulls have been found in the ruins of Pompeii. But 2,000 years later, the external features of these breeds have been radically altered and the sad truth is that many of these dogs are now suffering. Their facial anatomy has been significantly compressed to create a flatter and squarer skull shape, and their nostrils are narrow and resistant to airflow. The end of their palate is often overly long, obstructing the back of their throat. Their tongues are usually too large for their short faces. All of this results in snorting noises when they breathe, sleep apnoea, reduced ability to exercise, gut issues secondary to constantly gasping in air, and even a complete inability to breathe, which can result in a sudden and dramatic death.

I have heard Frenchies' and Bulldogs' breathing being likened to a human pinching their nose, breathing through a straw and running a marathon on a hot summer's day, and I think that's a pretty accurate description. Often, owners are not even aware of their issues. I have spoken to owners many times who feel that their dog has a perfectly good life with no breathing ailments, 'other than the snorting noise' (this is not normal), as long as they are kept quiet and not overly stimulated (again, not normal). Frenchie, devastatingly, is one of many dogs I see like this every week. A result of years of selective breeding has caused an epidemic of suffering. Well done us. We have produced a breed of flat-faced, squashed-skulled, bulging-eyed, short-jawed, aesthetically pleasing but desperately struggling canines and all because we think their faces look cuter that way. And their breathing issues are just part of myriad other health concerns. They are prone to eye ulcers due to the bulging prominent position of their eyeballs. Their excessive skin folds can become inflamed and infected. They often have malaligned jaws and suffer severe dental disease making picking up and eating food difficult. They have been bred with screw-shaped tails and thus frequently suffer from spinal disease. They are often unable to give birth naturally and require caesareans due to their narrow pelvis. A recent study found that more than 80% of Boston Terriers, Bulldogs and French Bulldogs are born by caesarean section.

When Miss Edmondson brought Frenchie in this morning, she mentioned to me that had she understood the issues of his breed before she'd purchased him – for the grand sum of £800 online – she would never have proceeded with the sale. And bang – there lies the heart of the issue. It has been estimated by vets across the UK that 75% of clients who own brachycephalic breeds are unaware of their potential health problems before deciding which type of dog to buy. Appearance is distressingly being placed as the number one priority over health. A further complicating factor is that brachycephalic dogs with chronic breathing difficulties often don't show the classic signs of pain, such as reduced appetite or subdued demeanour, that animals with other diseases may show. Many brachycephalic dog owners are keen advocates of animal welfare. They love their pet and want the best for them just as much as any other owner. Their Pugs and Frenchies are often friendly and excitable and are living life to the best degree they are able to, making their noisy breathing seem less significant. It can therefore come as a shock when vets question owners' choice of breed or express concern about their dog's quality of life. No one wants to feel judged and I can understand why this might discourage owners from bringing their dog to the vets. But from a welfare perspective it also makes educating people about the issues related to these breeds very difficult.

Adding fuel to the fire, owners are also being hit with extremely large vet bills to pay for the surgery and medical treatment required to maintain and improve their flat-faced dogs' lifestyles. Unfortunately, this means we are now seeing increasing numbers of brachycephalics abandoned at rehoming centres. The severity and volume of BOAS cases has caused vets across the UK finally to speak out and welfare groups, including the veterinary charities, The Kennel Club and even some breeders, are now making a stand against it.* When vets are slandered for trying to make money out of airway surgery on brachycephalic dogs, it makes me sad and rather angry. No vet anywhere wants an animal to suffer. Yes, we benefit financially from their condition as a profession, that is the nature of the beast, just like dentists make money from tooth decay and doctors on Harley Street benefit from women's infertility. But given the chance we would much rather it was never a requirement to operate on these dogs in the first place.

* An online platform to encourage vets to join the fight against breeding brachycephalics was launched in 2018 called Vets Against Brachycephalism. The British Veterinary Association (BVA) has created a #breedtobreathe campaign to promote choosing health over looks. The previous president of the BVA, Sean Wesley, has made a plea for prospective dog owners to 'consider the health harms perpetuated in dogs by purchasing brachycephalic breeds and choose a healthier alternative breed, or cross-breed instead'. The House of Lords has also called for people to 'respect animals as they are'.

I eventually walked away from Frenchie's kennel feeling deflated and knowing that I would be waking up tomorrow to do it all again.

26 SEPTEMBER 2014

Most weeks I get a message from a friend, or a friend of a friend, asking for advice about their pets' health. I don't tend to mind as it's all part of the job and it doesn't usually take me long to reply. The majority of the time my answer is some variation of the same theme: take your pet to your local vet to get him checked out if his or her symptoms don't improve.

Today's message was a bit different, and my standard reply didn't quite seem right.

'The guinea pig I've been looking after for a neighbour has died suddenly. Any ideas why? What should I do with the body?'

Having consulted my crystal ball to ascertain causes of death but found no answers, I replied to my friend with various options of what she could do with the body. She replied a little while later. 'The corn snake from the same family has now also escaped. Any ideas where it could have gone?'

Back to the crystal ball . . .

30 SEPTEMBER 2014

I saw Winnie today. Winnie belongs to Esther, our animal welfare officer. It's never easy treating staff animals, not least when they have had the kind of bumpy start to life that Winnie had. Everyone in the hospital is very attached to Winnie because of her story and the amount of time she has spent with us over the years. She was brought into the hospital in 2010, initially as a twelve-week-old puppy with a fracture of her right tibia (shin bone). Her owner, a young man in his twenties called Mr Brockbank, claimed he had been throwing Winnie in the air and he had missed when he tried to catch her. We treated the fracture, but five months later Mr

Brockbank brought her back again with concerns that she was not moving or eating and had a swollen right hind leg, the same leg as her previous injury. Mr Brockbank claimed there was no history of trauma and that he had no idea how Winnie had become this unwell. Sure enough, on examination she had swelling from the top of her right hind leg right down to her foot. She was dull, lacklustre and skinny. She is a medium-sized tan-coloured Staffie cross-breed and should have been in the prime of her life, but her muscles were wasting away, her bones jutting out at the hips and across her spine, and she appeared drawn and exhausted. She had two deep infected wounds around her mouth and her sad little face seemed to be silently willing us to help her. If only our patients could speak.

We admitted her for immediate veterinary care as she was in shock and a great deal of pain. The team worked together as we always do to save her life and make her as comfortable as possible, but none of us were prepared for the level of injuries we were about to discover on her X-rays. We started with the sore swollen leg. We found a fractured thigh bone and a hip bone fractured in several places. We went on to take X-rays of her chest, spine, pelvis, forelimbs and abdomen. She had fractured six ribs, her pelvis, her shoulder, her right front leg, both hips and her spine in several places. All fractures showed different stages of healing so we knew they had occurred over varying periods of time. She was completely unable to extend her back legs. In total we counted at least twenty fractures. She had digesting bony material in her stomach from scavenging or an inappropriate diet, and damage and bleeding at the back of one of her eyes, likely due to trauma.

News about Winnie spread around the hospital like wildfire. A second opinion from a specialist referral practice confirmed that the fractures were very unlikely to have occurred due to disease. We were dealing with a physical abuse case, the worst one I have seen so far in my career and possibly the worst one I will ever see. The degree of trauma required to fracture that number of bones, not just once but multiple times over many months, was unimaginable. The fear and suffering she must have endured over such a lengthy period was beyond comprehension. She was seized by the RSPCA under our recommendation and thankfully not allowed to return to her owner until after her case had been settled. Hopefully, never.

Heartbreakingly, several neighbours came forward following the RSPCA visit and reported having seen Mr Brockbank kicking Winnie regularly. In the early days after she came to us, the nurses worked around the clock to gently massage her legs, feed her, walk her, give her medications and try to persuade her that human beings weren't all bad. At various stages every vet in the hospital was involved in her care. We tried and failed to stay detached. Initial discussions included euthanasia as a possibility as her pain and suffering seemed too much. After several weeks, however, it became clear that Winnie was a determined and stoic fighter and despite the agony she must have experienced, she wanted to live. The entire hospital was rooting for her; we had to give her a chance. She underwent surgery on both hips and was started on heavy-duty painkillers which she would need to take every day for the rest of her life. But nothing would ever take her physical pain away completely, or fix the mental scars that would continue to haunt her.

Winnie was very wary of people and would lash out at strangers. She became particularly intolerant of vets, understandably, as we tended to prod and poke her where it hurt the most. But soon after she arrived, Esther began spending time with her and Winnie warmed to her immediately. Esther's other pets, her Jack Russell Terrier and her two cats, became Winnie's allies and before long Esther was fostering Winnie at her home. We all watched as this broken wreck of a dog started, little by little, to live the life she deserved. A life filled with love and companionship, tennis balls and treats, long walks across muddy fields and cuddles under the duvet. The depth of her bond with Esther was obvious for all to see. She trusted Esther with every fibre of her being. Esther had saved her, and they became inseparable.

Distressingly, Winnie's case never made it to court. Mr Brockbank, a drug addict known to the local authorities, was evicted from several properties during the initial few months Winnie was under RSPCA care. He eventually went off the radar. The RSPCA served an abandonment notice to his last known address, which he never responded to. We all waited with baited breath as the days ticked by, hoping he would not get in touch at the last moment. Thankfully, we heard no word from him and at the end of that notice period, six months after Winnie had escaped her life of torment, she was finally and permanently free. The only compensation for the trauma she had endured and the fact that Mr Brockbank would never be punished for his crimes was the fact that Winnie and Esther could now stay together for the rest of her days.

This brings us to today. Winnie and I have developed a love-hate relationship over the years. I love her and she hates me. I greatly look forward to seeing her and hearing what mischief she's been up to. But Winnie thinks I am a scrub-wearing devil in disguise. Winnie is usually lying on the floor being cuddled and caressed by multiple nurses when I see her. Today was no exception. As I walked into the room, her eyes met mine and the low growl was immediately audible. Her nurse fans left the room and Esther handled Winnie like a pro, muzzled and well held. Unfortunately, Winnie's extreme separation anxiety means that she has to accompany Esther to work every day on the train. Even more unfortunately, this resulted in liquid diarrhoea being squirted all across the train platform at rush hour this morning. After examining her and establishing that she'd most likely picked up a bug and reassuring Esther that she should be better within a few days, we parted ways until the next time. I watched Winnie totter down the corridor beside her and had a flashback to the terrified skinny trembling creature I had first met all those years ago and felt a sudden rush of emotion. What an unlucky dog to have ended up with Mr Brockbank. But what a lucky dog to have fallen into Esther's lap. I'm not sure I believe in fate, but if it does exist then this is what it must look like.

18 OCTOBER 2014

Went to my local pet food shop with James this morning to buy some food for Bea. I thought it was about time I started to practise what I preach after several years of buying whatever was on offer at the local supermarket, so off we went to investigate the different brands of quality cat food. I stood looking somewhat confused as James picked up various products and tried to mask his disappointment when I looked at them blankly and muttered something about good-quality protein.

'OK, but how does that translate into which brand to buy?' he asked.

'Um . . .' I stuttered, trying to retrieve some of the brief but essential information I was taught about nutrition at university from the recesses of my mind. 'Crude protein! Percentages! Obligate carnivores! We need to do away with all the crap carbohydrates,' I came out with, triumphantly.

James, looking unconvinced, started to do his own reading while I became distracted on the two-for-one packets of Dreamies aisle. Dreamies (second to catnip) are the crack of the cat world. Small balls of cheesy meaty feline deliciousness that have made a cat food company out there a LOT of money.

As I approached the counter area, I could hear Nigel, the pet food shop owner, chatting to another customer about her new Chihuahua puppy, Tinkerbell. Nigel, who had owned the shop for several decades and was a friendly amiable sort of chap, caught my eye and nodded hello to me. I smiled back. We had exchanged small talk many times about pet food and about my semi-savage big-haired feline flatmate. The lady he was chatting to continued on as she caressed Tinkerbell, who sat in her arms donning a large pink bow on her collar and hand-knitted red tartan dog jumper.

'. . . and the vet told me that it was perfectly fine to take Tinkerbell out to mix with other dogs at nine weeks old, despite not having been vaccinated,' she complained. 'Can you believe that! And they wanted to charge me two hundred and fifty pounds to have her neutered. Two hundred and fifty pounds!! I could go on holiday for that! And then they said she would need a micro-chip and a flea treatment and goodness knows what else. And your flea treatments here are half the price!'

Oh no, a vet-bashing session. I beat a hasty retreat and resisted the temptation to comment on the fact that veterinary-licensed flea treatments are expensive because they are safe and actually work, or that microchipping is a total no brainer. Why risk losing your dog or having her stolen with no way of finding her ever again?* I turned back to the aisles and continued in my pursuit of a decent brand of cat food. Ten minutes later, the lady had finished her rant and marched out of the shop with a disgruntled look on her face. I looked over to Nigel and gave him a little shrug.

'Oh dear, she didn't look happy,' I said.

'No. These vets. They are a strange bunch,' he replied.

'Hehe,' I laughed nervously. Did Nigel remember that I am a vet?

'They're always giving the wrong advice. Honestly, the number of times I've heard them saying awful things to owners. Don't they realise they are in a position of responsibility? And the amount they charge is just not reasonable.'

Was it too late to run out of the door and hide? Damn it, James was blocking the exit. I was going to have to respond.

'Um, yes. Do you remember I am a vet, Nigel? I see your point, and there are certainly some vets who give poor advice or over-charge but, in my experience, we are a fairly caring, responsible, well-informed bunch. Perhaps that lady got the wrong end of the stick with regard to the vaccination advice?' I offered, trying to stay neutral. Every vet

*From 6 April 2016 it was made compulsory for owners to ensure their dog is microchipped. Those who don't comply can be fined up to £500.

learns pretty close to day one at vet school that puppy vaccinations are recommended to prevent deadly viruses such as parvovirus and that until they have had a complete course of vaccinations, going on the floor or sniffing around other dogs' bottoms is not recommended.* The chances of a vet telling an owner that vaccinations aren't important and to throw a puppy straight into a ring of viral-infested adult dogs in a local park was extremely slim.

Nigel continued as if I hadn't spoken. He directed his next comment towards James. 'You must be aware that vets are an odd bunch, especially being married to one!'

James was avoiding eye contact and hastily paying for the cat food by this stage.

'You really wouldn't believe some of the stories I've heard. And it's true, they do charge an arm and a leg for flea products and for basic treatments!'

'Yes, I suppose we can be a bit of a strange breed, but we try our best!' I heard myself muttering as I backed out of the door. It was a Saturday and I wasn't in the mood for a debate. 'Bye then!'

I moaned to James for the entire walk home. I think he probably stopped listening about half way back, which was pretty good going. I really liked Nigel and it bothered me that he thought so little of the veterinary profession. I could usually tell which clients were going to go on a vet-bashing rant, but I hadn't seen it coming from him. I'd thought we were allies. There has been a great deal of press coverage recently about the prices that vets charge, and whether we are ultimately dishonest, untrustworthy, profit-focused businessmen and women. It makes me so sad. In one article I read, the author complained that the most common question asked by vets is, 'Are you insured?' I felt defensive of my veterinary

*Parvovirus is a nasty and ubiquitous bug passed through faeces that essentially punches holes in dogs' intestines and causes a rapid painful death. There is no cure and it can kill adult dogs as well as juvenile dogs. I have seen a 45kg two-year-old Rottweiler arrive dead at the clinic from parvovirus within twenty-four hours of developing symptoms.

community when I read this. I'm fairly certain that the hopes and dreams of new graduates do not include becoming a vet whose primary concern is insurance. But, in reality, part of our job description involves issuing bills and dealing with money whether we like it or not. In America, and most other countries in the world who do not have our beloved NHS, it is standard practice for doctors to ask if their patients are insured. This doesn't mean they don't care about them, but simply that the treatment they provide is not free. So why are vets chastised and complained about so unceremoniously in the UK for simply trying to make a living?

Perhaps a small percentage of vets are money-focused and are not prioritising practising good, honest medicine. But the majority of us, as corny as it sounds, do it for the love of the animals. Obviously we have to make some money in the process. We all live in the real world and have bills and mortgages to pay and considering the cost of equipment, drugs, training and staff salaries (to name just a few overheads), veterinary fees are often entirely justified, as expensive as they may seem. Vets as a general rule would always rather opt for the path of best standard of care, not the path of greatest financial gain. If the two coalesce then it's a win-win situation, but given the choice, many of us would rather not concern ourselves with bad debtors, bills and endless debates with owners about why our prices are so high.

I do understand why we are mistrusted. It must be difficult for members of the public who are not medically trained to appreciate why certain procedures are necessary, even when we have tried our best to explain it. When I take my car to the mechanic, if they tell me that the 'discombobulator' needs replacing and it is going to cost £1,000, I usually nod my head in mild confusion, have a small weep inwardly, do a frantic google search to try and understand what they are telling me, and then hand over my credit card. All I can do is hope and pray that they are being honest. And the same is true in the vet world. When your cat has a wound on his leg and you are told it will cost £600 to anaesthetise, treat and medicate him, it must seem absurdly expensive. When your dog has cancer and you are told you have to hand over £2,000 for surgery and chemo or he will die within the next few months, how do you know if this is true? Or whether this is the best path to follow? Should you follow the advice of the person in front of you? The only answer is trust. And if the trust isn't there, try another vet, or another, until you believe that the person standing in front of you is being honest. And if we are all saying the same thing, chances are it's because it's true.

1 NOVEMBER 2014

Just finished a busy on-call shift. We always receive calls around this time of year related to firework phobias and today was no exception. Many clients also came to their appointments today dressed in Halloween costumes on their way out to Saturday night Halloween parties, which was entertaining, although there is something disconcerting about discussing a dog's euthanasia with a man dressed as the murderer from *Scream*, complete with a (hopefully fake) knife in hand.

After a quick selfie with my colleagues who had finished their shifts and were off out to their own Halloween parties dressed as zombies in scrubs and fake blood, I jumped on to reception to answer some calls. This happens rarely as usually the reception team are handling the calls themselves, and the vets are pretty rubbish at dealing with the admin side of things. I often fail at the first hurdle, such as knowing which benefits make a client eligible for our treatment (this information seems to vary all the time), which details our clients are required to bring to their appointment with them, or how to process a donation through a client's file over the phone. I genuinely believe that the receptionists have one of the most difficult jobs in the hospital. They are the face of PWH, the first staff clients come across when they enter or call the hospital. They are expected to answer medical questions related to booking appointments when they have received little or no medical training. They are also expected to be polite and knowledgeable at all times regardless of the type of query or unpleasant attitude of some of the clients. Frequently I have heard the reception team being shouted at or threatened because they have asked for a contribution towards their pet's treatment or to see a client's benefit details. Then that same client has come through into my consulting room to see me with a sweet smile on their face as if nothing has happened. Some days I know they receive abuse relentlessly and yet they soldier on and still try their best to do their jobs with a smile on their faces.

This afternoon, we were short staffed and the phone was ringing non-stop. When I took my first call I crossed my fingers it would be a medical question and not a technical or eligibility-related one.

'PWH emergency line, how can I help you?' I asked.

'My dog is stuck to my wardrobe by her eyeball,' a female voice mumbled at the other end of the phone.

'Excuse me?' I asked, confused. Maybe I hadn't heard correctly. Or maybe it was some kind of Halloween practical joke?

'My Bichon, Daisy, was terrified by the noise of fireworks. She went crazy running about and ran straight into the wardrobe. But it's one of those temporary ones with a zip at the front, and she somehow got her eye stuck to the zip bit and I can't get it off!'

The client sounded panicked, understandably. I could hear poor Daisy whimpering in the background. After asking a few more questions I established that Daisy had been seen by us recently for a weight check and was a healthy ten-year-old dog, apart from her obesity and the wardrobe stuck to her face. With a little more investigating I managed to find out that the wardrobe itself was made of a polyester material and I encouraged the client – whose name was Miss Beddington – to find some scissors and attempt to cut Daisy free.

'Obviously try to keep the scissors far away from her face. You're not trying to cut the eyelashes or eyelid, just the material attached to the main part of the wardrobe so you can bring her in to us,' I explained, fearful that Miss Beddington may misunderstand my instructions and start attempting some sort of heroic eye surgery.

Eventually, after disappearing away from the phone for several minutes, Miss Beddington returned and assured me that she had managed to free her dog with unharmed eyeball still in situ. Hurrah! Forty minutes later they arrived at the hospital. Sure enough, poor fat Daisy walked in with a large bouffant white curly hairdo and a piece of wardrobe sticking out of her face, attached via a zip on to the fleshy part of her eyelid, while Miss Beddington was dressed as a witch with a tall black hat and make-up streaming down her face where she had been crying. They made quite a pair.

I admitted Daisy straight away for emergency surgery. Remarkably, once she was under anaesthetic and I was able to assess her properly, I could see that she had managed to avoid damage to the eyeball itself, which under the circumstances was nothing short of a miracle. Using wire cutters, I cut through the metal part of the zip, being careful not to cause further damage to her eyelid, and it instantly broke apart and detached. I breathed out loudly and realised I had been holding my breath. She had a deep slice through her inner eyelid but it should heal up. What a lucky little fluffy lady she was. I called the owner after the surgery and she was extremely relieved and tearful. I encouraged her to consider firework anxiety desensitisation therapy using CDs with firework noises the following year and to try sedative drugs this year to get Daisy through the next few days. I also recommended she purchase a new wardrobe, preferably one without zips. Her current one now had a large dog-shaped hole in it, after all.

I hung the phone up and couldn't help but smile. Every time I think I have encountered all possible scenarios and nothing else can shock or amuse me, something does. It's a big part of why I love this job. Always expect the unexpected, especially at Halloween.

3 NOVEMBER 2014

Had an emergency call from a friend tonight who lives across the road. I affectionately refer to her as 'crazy-but-lovely neigh-bour'. Her cat had brought in a mouse, what was she supposed to do now? I detected from the hint of hysteria in her voice that she needed some skilled veterinary assistance. I ran over, Tupperware in hand, to find my friend tucked under a blanket on her sofa with her kids, hiding from the fiendish mouse. I used my best vet skills to thrust the cat in one direction and flip the Tupperware over said mouse as it whizzed across the carpet. After reassuring the kids that mice are lovely little things, look at his sweet little face, etc., I ran back to salvage my burning dinner, with a quick stop-off in the garden to release the alarmed but surprisingly unharmed looking mouse. All in a day's work.

6 NOVEMBER 2014

Had a hospital appointment today with a surgeon about a minor procedure I need to have. His bedside manner was interesting to say the least. What is it about human surgeons, particularly at consultant level, that makes them communicate in such a dismissive and brusque way with their patients? Is it the sheer volume of hours they have worked and the graft they have put in, combined with a sense of NHS-underfunded and overworked doom? Or did they all start out with a fatal inability to talk to other humans in a polite and chatty manner? Don't get me wrong, I think doctors are amazing, and those working in the NHS especially so. My father worked in the NHS for thirty years and my brother is now following suit, slogging his guts out as a junior doctor. But surgeons in particular are a funny breed. The man I met today is one of several surgeons I have met – both male and female – who seem to forget that there is a patient attached to the condition. You come across it in the vet world too. Vets who are incredibly talented surgeons and could name every part of every bone in the body of multiple species, but make clients feel about as relaxed during a consultation as they would on a trip to the morgue. I understand it slightly more with vets as there may have been a misconception from the start that this job is about animals and not about people. In fact, nothing could be further from the truth. The triangle of vet-patient-client can make it even more complicated ensuring communication is adequate, possibly akin only to paediatrics. 'Never work with children or animals' as the old saying goes.

I left the hospital after my appointment today, reminding myself to continue to cherish and enjoy the chit-chat I have with my clients and to never forget that despite the various challenges of my working day, every owner is just trying to make their story heard. The least I can do is make them feel listened to.

10 NOVEMBER 2014

Spent the day battling the elements in our mobile clinic van, which travels around London to access a wider client base. The chill in the air made my toes numb and both my colleague Tom, the van driver, and I were wrapped in thick generic blue fleeces, concealing our names and job titles. Cue: classic gender discrimination as Mrs Harris stepped on to the van with Harry her miniature Schnauzer and completely ignored me in preference for my male colleague who she assumed was the vet. Standard. Sadly and disappointingly, I have come across gender discrimination from clients on a regular basis since graduation. I find the old-fashioned concept of a male vet being more capable than his female counterpart, or the assumption that a man must be the one in the position of authority, pretty baffling. Even more so in light of the current 'feminisation' of the profession that is occurring across Britain and America. Eighty per cent of my year group at vet school were women.

You'd have thought the stethoscope around my neck would have given it away. Even when Tom and I corrected her, Mrs Harris still continued to address her concerns about Harry to him and not to me. It was only when I listened to Harry's heart and detected a murmur that needed investigating that she seemed remotely convinced I knew what I was talking about.* I was very tempted to pop across to a café and warm up over a cup of hot chocolate while Tom held the rest of the consultation, but I persisted with my examination. I even resisted the urge to make her wait two months for Harry's heart scan just so that she could see a male vet (who is an ophthalmologist, not a heart specialist, by the way) rather than booking her in to see me the following week.

13 NOVEMBER 2014

I seem to be suffering from hand-and-foot-in-mouth disease today. Just asked a client with one arm to give me a hand getting his dog on to the consultation table, shortly after asking the visually impaired client before him with a patch over one eye to keep an eye on her dog's lameness. Luckily, neither client took offence, or even seemed to notice me quietly dying inside.

17 NOVEMBER 2014

Mr King, the owner of an English Bulldog called Boris, came to see me in clinic today. It is unusual to maintain decent case continuity in charity practice because, in contrast to small rural practices where there may be only one or two vets and no other practices for miles around, we are hardly ever in the same place at the same time from one day to the next. With twelve permanent vets, various locums, three London branch practices, a mobile clinic that rotates around London, clinic shifts and surgical shifts, weekend and emergency work, I'm lucky if I can remember where I am meant to be each day, let alone see the same clients each week. Mr King was one of the few exceptions. I have known Boris since he

*A heart murmur is an additional abnormal heart sound that can be heard when listening to the heart with a stethoscope. It is caused by turbulent blood flow and often needs investigating to establish what it means for the animal.

was only one year old when he came to see me in 2008, shortly after I started working at PWH. I had had limited exposure at that stage to dealing with clients with significant mental health problems. They don't teach you much about this at university. Vet school is a bubble of academia and although universities are improving their communication training and now get actors in to play clients in various scenarios with the final year students, you still graduate with very limited experience of dealing with real people in real-life situations. So when Mr King, a young man in his twenties, walked through the door with a swagger, smelling of marijuana and with a disgruntled look on his face, I was immediately out of my depth.

The conversation began with a six-minute monologue about how none of us 'incompetent vets' had managed to fix his dog's skin disease. Poor Boris has atopy, a hereditary and life-long allergic skin condition which we see every day in first opinion practice, and is frustratingly often passed down through generations of dogs. It can cause alarming levels of itchiness, resulting in dogs ripping their skin to shreds in an attempt to satisfy the itch. There is sadly no quick fix and limited options for ongoing management in charity practice. The condition is at best tolerable and at worst unmanageable no matter what therapy we throw at them. In private practice and referral practices, management of atopy tends to focus on the search for, and if possible the elimination of, the cause of the flare-ups. Unfortunately, allergen-specific immunotherapy (a form of desensitisation to environmental allergies) and several other modern immune-suppressive drugs used to treat atopy are prohibitively expensive for most charity practices. Our clients require referral to a dermatologist if they wish to pursue these treatment options.

Mr King's complaint (which I surmised through the ranting) was that Boris had required several courses of antibiotics and steroids to help improve his symptoms and his quality of life, and yet here he was a month later itching and scratching and clearly not fixed. Apparently we don't care about animals either because we had asked to see his benefit details and for a contribution towards treatment at the previous visit. After examining Boris, a sweet dopey boy with sad eyes and red-raw skin, I set about the task of explaining gently to Mr King that he had missed his recheck appointment two weeks ago and that stopping his medication suddenly had caused the skin condition to flare up again. I tried to explain that Boris has a chronic condition which would require ongoing treatment and regular check-ups throughout his life. I mentioned referral to a specialist and explained what this would cost. This merely angered Mr King more. The icing on the cake came when I broached the subject of castration and explained the potentially hereditary nature of the disease.

'Any puppies he fathered would be at risk of developing similar skin issues,' I said gently. 'And being a charity we don't promote breeding anyway.'

At this stage, Mr King began shouting an escalating series of obscenities, terminating in the delightful threat that if I tried to remove Boris's 'nuts', he would be waiting for me after work to 'cut me up'.

Luckily, or possibly unluckily, my consulting-room door was open and another client overheard this. Very soon there was a rowdy dispute occurring in which the second client was threatening Mr King, saying that her boyfriend would be escorting me to the tube station that evening and would deal with Mr King herself.

Oh God.

I quickly closed the door to separate them, made eye contact with my head receptionist who had come to check I was OK and gave her a nod to say I was fine. My heart was thumping in my chest but I tried to maintain an air of dignified calm as I attempted to bring the consultation down a notch. I was reluctant to leave and ask someone else to take over because somehow that would feel like he had won. I refused to let him intimidate me. I straightened myself up, all five-foot-three of me, and looked up to the six-foot bulky man standing in front of me.

'Mr King. Please be aware that any threats to staff members

will not be tolerated and you will not be seen back here again in the future if you continue to behave in this way. As I have explained, we have several options for Boris that will help us to manage his skin problem, but we need to work together. We are not trying to be difficult or to upset you in any way. We are all working towards the same goal, which is to make Boris's life as comfortable as possible. Now please have the patience to listen to what I have to say.'

He seemed to appreciate the frankness and surprisingly stepped back and leaned against the wall while I continued to talk him through my suggested approach to Boris's skin issues. Even more surprisingly, he eventually apologised to me for being, in his own words, 'aggro'. He explained that he couldn't afford to keep coming back to the practice, that he had forty pence to his name (which he insisted on pulling out of his pocket to show me), that his mother was ill, his father was in prison and that he hadn't even wanted to take Boris on but had rescued him from another boy on his estate who was beating him. The consultation eventually came to a close and Mr King headed down to dispensary to collect Boris's medication. He left no donation and I have no doubt that Boris went on to father countless puppies that are currently wandering around London with their inherited skin disease. However, I still felt proud of myself for not running out of the room and hiding under a table.

I have since seen Mr King and Boris back every year for the same recurrent skin issues and today was no different. Boris is seven years old now and the skin over his paws and abdomen is chronically thickened and scarred from countless flare-ups of his condition. Rather bizarrely, I have developed a bit of a soft spot for both Boris and Mr King now and he has been unexpectedly civil to me since our initial altercation. We have reached some sort of equilibrium and these days he even attempts to stick to appointment times and leaves small contributions towards treatment.

The Mr King incident is an example of one of the hundreds of threats received by me and other staff members from clients at

PWH every year, and unfortunately charity practice is not unique in this regard. A survey by the BVA found that nearly 90% of UK vets have experienced some form of intimidation including swearing, shouting and threats of violence. 60% of vets claim to experience this sort of behaviour at least every couple of months, while almost a third at least monthly and 13% daily. Sadly, but unsurprisingly the survey also showed that women and younger vets were significantly more likely to be threatened. In private practice, many of these cases are related to the cost of treatment. In charity practice, although finances are less of an issue with respect to the client-vet interaction, we still have our own set of challenges. Our clients have often led difficult lives and are fighting against their own demons. I try very hard to remember this when confronted with the 'Mr Kings'. Everyone can have a bad day. People can become angry because they love their pets and are afraid, but that doesn't necessarily make them a bad person. Of course, that doesn't justify aggressive behaviour, but it does make it easier for me to tolerate being on the receiving end of it on a regular basis. Despite his anger-management issues, Mr King was essentially just a young man who had been dealt a pretty rough hand in life and was worried about his dog. Some issues are definitely down to an individual vet's approach to their clients, that's for sure. Not every personality type will get along, but facing situations with a positive mental attitude and a lack of judgement certainly helps. I have found that being a vet and being exposed daily to clients from all walks of life offers a unique view of humankind and society in general. It's a mixed bag. Where there is someone unreasonable, someone reasonable will follow. There is rarely a purely lovely or purely nasty client. People can be complex and flawed and interesting and resilient and irritating and brilliant all at once. Society, after all, is filled with good people, bad people, and then most of the rest of us who lie somewhere in between.

19 NOVEMBER 2014

Newsflash to all owners out there: testing sugar levels in urine samples to check for diabetes is pretty ineffectual when a urine sample has been brought in in an unwashed honey pot. And while we are on this topic, that also goes for jam jars, sweet jars, sugar jars and generally anything that once had food or edible liquids in it. Or non-edible liquids. Or non-edible solids come to that. Basically – just use the urine pot provided.

20 NOVEMBER 2014

Just finished a consultation about a dog's diet who is being fed Chappie – a commercially available common brand of dog food containing either fish, beef or chicken mixed with cereals or rice. It is cheap and cheerful and comes out of the tin in large clumps of meatiness that dogs seem to love. I can report from experience that it barely looks any different when it comes out again the other end.

Me: So what are you feeding Sammy?

Ms Hardy: Chappie. It's great, he's been on it for a few months now. I wanted him to be vegan like me.

Me: OK . . . But are you aware that Chappie is not a vegan food?

Ms Hardy: Yes it is.

Me: Um . . . no, I'm pretty sure it contains meat or fish products.

Ms Hardy: No it doesn't.

Me: OK, well either way, Sammy is an omnivore like us so actually this diet will be perfect for him as he needs a mixture of meat, carbohydrate and vegetables to get all the vitamins and minerals he requires.

Ms Hardy: Well, I thought it was vegan. Just rice. That's annoyed me now. I want him to eat vegan food. So what else can I give him then?

Me: Well, I wouldn't recommend a vegan diet for dogs to be honest. But if you really want to give him one then you will have to do a fair amount of research. The best way to ensure he's getting the correct nutrients is to feed him dog food rather than a home-cooked vegan diet. The trouble is that many of the commercially available vegetarian diets also have fish oils in them so they aren't actually vegan. If you cook for him at home you will need to replace his protein from somewhere. Maybe consider soya bean or quinoa? Although quinoa isn't cheap. Plus he may not find them palatable and they may cause flatulence, so be careful.

Ms Hardy: What are those things?

Me: Soya and quinoa are alternative sources of protein.

Ms Hardy: OK, or what about plain pasta?

Me: Pasta is fine as an additional carbohydrate, but not ideal as a meat replacement.

Ms Hardy: OK, so maybe some rice with the pasta?

Me: Again, a good source of carbohydrate but not a good meat substitute. You want to replace the iron and protein that meat usually provides, so maybe something like lentils or beans?

Ms Hardy: Oh, I see. [Pauses. Nods head as if deep in thought.] What about herbs then?

Me: . . .

I admire her determination but I dread to think what Ms Hardy is feeding herself let alone poor Sammy. Pasta with rice and a side portion of parsley, anyone?

23 NOVEMBER 2014

Most veterinary practices have a 'practice pet', usually a three-legged cat or a one-eyed rabbit or maybe even a bald stray hamster. At PWH our 'practice pet', who is actually owned by one of the senior nurses, Sophie, is a ginger cat called Diego. Diego is a very special boy. He commutes into work each day with her in a cat carrier on the train, happy as Larry, people watching, reading the *Metro* and snoozing. He even has his own travel card. He spends his days in our cat ward at the hospital chilling out, playing with toys and being showered with love by all the nurses. It may sound curious that a cat would tolerate this sort of lifestyle, but Diego is paraplegic. He was born with spina bifida. *

In addition to her day job at PWH, Sophie helped to set up an animal charity called New Hope Animal Rescue. She's a modern Doctor Doolittle, often working through the night to care for the animals at New Hope, many of whom live with her in her actual house, after doing a full day's shift at PWH. She does everything in her power to save the animals who are lucky enough to find their way to her, and Diego was no exception. He was rescued by Sophie when he was only six weeks old after the owner signed him over to New Hope. The condition had left him with almost completely paralysed hindlimbs and they no longer wanted him because of his disability. When I first examined him, he resembled a small ball of ginger fluff with back legs that splayed out behind him like a frog. He moved his back legs weakly in a swimming motion although his front end was completely normal and he played with his toys like any other kitten. He had an inquisitive and expressive little face and it was absolutely impossible not to love him.

Following referral to a neurologist and a diagnosis of spina bifida, Sophie decided it was kindest to consider putting him to sleep. But Diego seemed extremely content despite his disability and within a short period of time he had found a way to move around and enjoy life. Each time Sophie went to put him to sleep she changed her mind at the last minute and despite animal

---

*Spina bifida is a condition that occurs in humans and animals where the bones of the vertebrae (spine) don't form properly around the spinal cord. In Diego's case this defect was very severe so the nerves running down his spinal cord failed to connect to his back legs and also affected his bladder control.

welfare being my upmost priority, I had to agree with her that he seemed a pretty happy little chap. Most days, vets question themselves at least once about an animal's quality versus quantity of life. It's a hugely important aspect of our job. Television programmes such as *The Supervet*, which demonstrates bionic inventions and prosthetic limbs on animals as tiny as rabbits, have shown animal medicine in a whole new light. There is a new world of possibility for our pets and what was previously 'the end' could now simply mark a new beginning. But the question that lingers in my mind is – just because we can, does this mean we should? Diego could be kept alive and cared for, but should he be? What constitutes a life worth living?

Essentially it often comes down to the subjective opinions of the vets and nurses caring for the animal in question rather than a blanket rule for all. Medicine is so rarely black and white. On paper, Diego sounded like an animal that was suffering, but in reality I had never before encountered a cat with his sort of relaxed demeanour. Nothing seemed to faze him. He hadn't known any other life so he contentedly got on with the one he'd been given. Sophie's dedication to his care was extraordinary. He slept on her pillow next to her every single night and continues to do so to this day. It quickly became apparent that his quality of life was very good. In fact, he was pretty much leader of the pack back at home, a pack that included fifteen dogs, five cats, four rabbits, three 200kg pigs and a handful of turkeys and chickens. It's safe to say that Diego had challenged my understanding of the term 'quality of life'. He was happier and more fulfilled than many able-bodied cats I had come across. In another situation where a kitten like Diego had not landed on the doorstep of a qualified and committed veterinary nurse, or had had a feisty temperament and appeared unhappy with a life spent being cared for by a human, the outcome would have been very different.

Today I saw Diego in clinic for a check-up. I examined him in all his ginger glory. At the age of eight months he was now a little ginger lion but had retained his kitten-like baby face. His top end was completely normal, bright eyed, curious, full of life. His back legs were weak and skinny from the muscle wastage, but he sat purring away happily on the table, occasionally batting a fluffy ball that was hanging from the end of my pen. Sometimes I think we could all learn a thing or two from Diego. He lives his life to the fullest. What a dude.

24 NOVEMBER 2014

Had a student in theatre with me today watching me do a bitch spay. We usually only allow veterinary medicine students in their clinical years into the operating theatre. I spent about twenty minutes during the op explaining in intricate detail to her what I was doing.

'Now I am gently placing traction on the ovarian ligament.'

'Now I am breaking apart the mesometrium and making a window with my tissue forceps.'

'Now I am placing my second ligature around the ovarian vessels, using a polyfilament material. We can discuss the pros and cons of the different suture materials later if you like.'

She seemed a little quiet. I thought she might just be shy. Eventually she piped up and spoke just as I was finishing my surgery. 'What's a spay?' she asked.

'Um, it's the surgery I have just been doing to remove a dog's uterus and ovaries. What year are you in at vet school again?'

'Oh no, I'm not at vet school. I'm in year nine. I'm fourteen. I'm just here to help in kennels but it was quiet so they sent me up here.'

Note to self: always check age of audience before imparting pearls of surgical wisdom.

25 NOVEMBER 2014

I saw a puppy for his vaccinations this afternoon that was registered as a Dalmatian. When the owner brought him in it quickly became clear that he was, in fact, a Staffie with white and black spots.

'Where did you get Max from then, Mr Perkins?'

'We purchased him for six hundred pounds from an online breeder.'

Oh dear. People buying dogs online has become a pet hate of mine, pardon the pun. I have no idea how or why it is legal to sell animals on the Internet but unfortunately it is. Every vet knows the story about the client who brought their new black and tan Rottweiler puppy in to be seen by a vet for the first time, only to find out they had actually spent hundreds of pounds purchasing a black and tan guinea pig. But far worse than that, I have seen puppies and kittens brought into the hospital in dire conditions, covered in diarrhoea, skinny and dying of flea anaemia and preventable viruses, more often over the years I have been in charity practice than I care to remember. Countless times I have been called over to the emergency room at two or three in the morning on a night shift to treat little Chihuahua or Yorkshire Terrier puppies that have been sold online by backyard breeders. They are almost always undersized, having been ripped away from their mother and litter mates too early, and too small and fragile to maintain their blood sugar levels. They arrive semi-comatose in a state of shock, with diarrhoea matted around their back ends. They are often terrified and very poorly and the owners, who have tried their best to do the right thing, are already attached to their new pet and also deeply distressed. Sometimes these puppies survive and go on to have emotional issues related to being removed from their family too soon, but sometimes they die painfully and unnecessarily. Very rarely have the owners seen the mother of the puppy they have purchased, let alone the father, litter mates or the conditions of the breeding unit, if you can call it that.

Many times, owners have reported to me that the 'deal' took place on the side of a road and by the time they realised that the puppy was not very well and that the breeder was unlikely to be bona fide, it was too late and they just wanted to rescue the puppy from its current environment. Owners rarely have the details of the breeder or a working telephone number that could be given to the police or RSPCA and, even more worryingly, the police are afraid to visit the travelling sites where they are being bred even if details were made available. According to Dogs Trust, who have performed several investigations into the illegal entry of dogs into the UK, many dogs are also being brought in illegally from puppy farms in eastern Europe and Ireland to supply the market for brachycephalic breeds like French Bulldogs. The controls at UK border ports appear to be ineffective. Dogs are being issued with false passports, and therefore are unlikely to be vaccinated against rabies, and many of them are entering the UK riddled with parasites. They are regularly sedated to allow them to be brought across the UK border without detection. The conditions of their transportation have been found to be squalid and cramped, often travelling for thirty hours with little water and no toilet breaks. Dogs Trust have reported that approximately six per cent of these puppies are dying either in transit or shortly after arrival. Heavily pregnant bitches are also being forced to travel on long gruelling journeys in order to reach the UK in time to give birth because UK born puppies are likely to sell quicker. Figures released by DEFRA revealed that the number of declared dogs entering the UK from Lithuania increased by 780% between 2011 and 2013 and by 663% from Hungary. Worryingly, this doesn't even include the number of dogs entering the UK illegally. With each illegally imported puppy being sold for an average of £1,400, the amount of money being made is now being compared to the drug trade.

The sale of pets online is an issue vets are silently battling but unable to control because currently there are simply no laws or restrictions on it in the UK.[*] Puppies can be purchased at the click of a button regardless of their age and health status or how poor the conditions of the breeding unit they have come from are. Educating owners about breeding, socialising and training their dogs is one of the main aspects of my job. But sadly so many people still ignore the advice vets give them and use dog ownership for illegal and irresponsible purposes. I deeply wish that there was more information available to help owners make more educated decisions about where and how to purchase a pet, but for now all we can do is try and spread the word within our small veterinary community.

If I were asked by a friend or family member where to get a pet from, I would suggest that they consider a rescue shelter first and foremost. Many animal charities, including the RSPCA, PDSA, Blue Cross, Dogs Trust and Cats Protection, now provide free advice on their websites about where to get a dog from and which pet might be right for them. The PDSA, for example, has a link on their website to a free 'Puppy Contract' and 'Puppy Information Pack', in addition to offering consultations for their clients to come and discuss the options before committing to a pet. If rehoming a rescue dog was not an option then I would tell them to look at the Kennel Club's list of registered breeders, or even local families whose pets have had a litter. I would highly recommend they visit the breeder's home to see with their own eyes what conditions the animals are being kept in, although even then you still have to be careful. Unscrupulous breeders will hide the

[*]As of 1 October 2018, the Animal Welfare Act of 2006 was amended so that people breeding and selling dogs for commercial gain in the UK must now have a special licence and are not permitted to sell dogs or cats under eight weeks of age. The government has recently announced plans to alter the law further so that animals less than six months old can only be purchased or adopted from a registered breeder or a rescue centre. It's a good start, but time will tell how well the changes will be implemented.

squalid filthy conditions they breed in at the back of their property, or sell their puppies and kittens through pet shops that look perfectly hygienic to unsuspecting customers. If there is any doubt, do not complete the purchase. See both the mother and father dogs if possible. Ask how many litters the mother dog has had and in what time-period. Seek official documentation on any vaccinations that have been administered and request passports if they have come from abroad. And finally, I would tell them that whatever route they go down, they must not purchase animals that are being bred as commodities and illegally imported or they will be involving themselves in a chain of animal cruelty that vets are trying desperately to fight against.

With all this whizzing through my mind, and with a sense of déjà vu, I started to examine Max. 'I'm not completely sure he is a pedigree Dalmatian,' I said gently. 'He looks like he could have some Staffordshire Bull Terrier in him.' (Around 90% at a guess, with the remaining 10% being pure mongrel.)

'Oh yes, he is definitely a Dalmatian. We have the paperwork for him and everything. And he's had his first vaccination and is flea treated.'

The owner produced a typed note that indeed claimed that the puppy had had his first vaccination already (there was no legally required veterinary vaccination card or signature to certify this), and that he was a ten-week-old male pedigree Dalmatian, and had been given a non-prescription flea treatment two weeks earlier.

I finished examining Max, who was absolutely gorgeous regardless of his breed. He was a tiny, skinny, pot-bellied ball of delight and one of the more healthy puppies from an online breeder I have encountered. I decided not to pursue the pedigree discussion as the owner seemed adamant about him being a Dalmatian, and what good would it do now anyway.

'I think we ought to start his vaccination programme from scratch,' I said. 'Without a vaccination certificate signed by a veterinary surgeon we can't be sure he had his first one. Better safe than sorry. Also, I'm pretty sure he isn't actually ten weeks old, so even if he did have it I think he would have been too young for it to take effect. I'd put him at about six or seven weeks.'

'Right, OK. He was the biggest in the litter,' Mr Perkins muttered. He was getting cross.

'I suspect unfortunately that he's been taken from his mum a bit too soon and I'm afraid to say he also has fleas. I suspect he might have worms too. But on the plus side he seems to be in robust health otherwise and we can easily treat the parasites.' I tried to reassure him despite unintentionally discrediting all the information on the letter from the breeder. 'I suggest we postpone the vaccine for another week or two until he's the right age.'

Now Mr Perkins was seriously fed up. I managed to get him back on side by giving Max an abundance of cuddles and complimenting his cute puppy face, ignoring the itchy sensation washing over me as I canoodled him and his creepy crawly pals.

The consultation was drawing to a close after a chat about general puppy care, diet and the perils of purchasing pets online. I think Mr Perkins was starting to understand that online puppy sellers often can't be trusted. I felt we had developed a bit of a rapport by this stage and repaired some of the damage done by my multiple revelations. He was just about to leave when I noticed something else.

'Oh, one more thing, Mr Perkins. He's actually a girl. How do you feel about the name Maxine?'

26 NOVEMBER 2014

A lovely but timid Staffie called Bubble came to see me on the mobile van today. She was brought in by an elderly lady, Mrs Heppell, and her younger neighbour. Mrs Heppell had been going about her usual business the night before when she'd heard Bubble barking in the back garden. She looked out of the window and saw a group of boys in their late teens encouraging

Bubble to stick her head through a gap in the fence. She did so and then got her head stuck. The boys (this was Mrs Heppell's descriptive term for them although they should more accurately be described as young men) then proceeded to beat Bubble around the face with sticks. Bubble was writhing and shrieking and barking as they continued their assault. As Mrs Heppell recounted this story she began visibly shaking and leaned against her neighbour, a kind-looking man in his fifties, for support. I put an arm around her and comforted her. She had been too frightened to go out and stop them so had had to stand and watch until her neighbour had luckily intervened and chased them off. He managed to free Bubble from the fence and returned her to Mrs Heppell, who was afraid to contact the police in case the 'boys' came after her.

Sadly, and all too familiar a story in this job, Bubble had come from a history of abuse already. Mrs Heppell had rescued her as a younger dog having spent the first two years of her life as a breeding bitch. She had been exposed to very little in the way of love or kindness from the humans around her. Despite this, she was trusting and allowed me to examine her fully. She was a medium-sized white Staffie with saggy teats from her years of rearing puppies. She had bruising and small puncture wounds all over her face and one large laceration to her chin that would require stitches. She wagged her tail but held her head low, slightly unsure of my intentions and seeking constant reassurance from her owner. I gave her a gentle stroke and then sent her off to our main hospital to be stitched up.

After she left I shook my head in frustration. I feel ashamed to belong to this species sometimes. What must Bubble think of humans after all she's experienced? Goodness knows what else those young men were capable of. Worryingly, all of the statistics seem to indicate that animal abuse is frequently the precursor to, or occurs alongside, child or spouse abuse. Much of the evidence linking animal abuse and domestic violence is from studies in the USA, although there is now a growing research base in the UK. The NSPCC produced a leaflet in 2005, with the support of many other services and charities including PWH, called 'Understanding the Links' that has been circulated around the UK to raise awareness about this issue among professionals. In the leaflet, they state that 'The relationship of a child and its family to its family pets will tell you a great deal, and should be included in any assessment of need.' It makes sense that people who are willing to harm a defenceless pet for no reason would do the same to a weaker family member, and vice versa.

As I stood contemplating this, a lady in her fifties with crooked teeth, mousey brown hair and a flowery outfit resembling some eighties curtains approached the mobile van.

'I'm so sorry but I had to buy a cup of tea because I used the loo in a café and then felt bad that I had used their facilities without buying anything, otherwise I would have had a whole five pounds!' she blurted out as if we were midway through a conversation. 'I work for an animal charity too – well, in their charity shop actually – and I always walk past your van and think I must donate, but these days I never have any spare change as I give all my spare pennies to them now!' She carried on without pausing for breath. 'My husband tells me I must accept the occasional bit of kindness from others as I like to give it all away, my money and my time that is, and I suppose he's right. Anyway, I'm off to the cemetery now to see if my flowers are still alive. I used to have lots of family around here, but not anymore. I wonder if they'll let me use their toilet when I get there. After the tea I'm sure to need it again. The facilities are terrible in that area!' And with that, she handed me £4.20 and disappeared before I even had a chance to thank her.

'I hope your flowers are still alive!' I called after her.

If it wasn't for the money in my hand I would have thought I had imagined the whole conversation. I popped her donation into our pot and smiled. It's a funny old world. So much badness, but thankfully so much goodness to counteract it.

27 NOVEMBER 2014

Me: How can I help you today?

Owner: I am so worried about Diana, she's got a big lump on her back. The kids will be devastated if anything happens to her. Please tell me there is something you can do for her.

Me: [Examines Diana, the fluffy lop-eared rabbit. Removes 'lump', aka boiled sweet attached to the fur on her back.]

Fixed!

28 NOVEMBER 2014

I had been looking forward to some drinks with colleagues after work last week. It's rare to make any solid plans, certainly none that start before 8 p.m. and my friends outside of work are used to me running late or cancelling last minute. The handy thing about making plans with other vets is that we are all as unreliable as each other. If we need to delay timings or cancel last minute because an emergency arrives as we are walking out of the door then no one is offended. We were doing well though and were almost good to go when I realised my colleague and good pal Sarah was still in theatre.

She was scrubbed into a leg amputation on an eight-month-old 30kg Husky puppy called Teddy that had been in a car accident two days earlier. Sadly, his leg fracture was too severe to be fixed and amputation was the only option. I stuck my head into theatre to see if all was OK. The room was tense. Sarah had almost finished the surgery but something wasn't right. The nurse on anaesthesia duty was scrambling around Teddy's chest trying to find a heartbeat. Teddy had had an unexpected cardiac arrest two hours into surgery and about five minutes before he would have been woken up.

In general practice in the UK, we rarely if ever work with a veterinary surgeon anaesthetist. In the event of an anaesthetic emergency, technically while the vet is busy with the surgery, they shouldn't allow the veterinary nurse to alter the anaesthetic settings without specific instructions to do so. This places both the nurse and vet in an impossible position and is one of the huge differences between human and animal surgery and anaesthesia in terms of staffing logistics and the limited resources that we have to work with. I rushed in to help and luckily my veterinary colleague Lucy and two other nurses also came to assist. I have heard veterinary anaesthesia described as 98% boredom and 2% panic and I don't think that's far from the truth. We were suddenly and unwelcomely thrust into our 2% panic moment and yet, due to the vast experience of the team I work with, everything remained remarkably calm. Phrases such as 'start breathing for him', 'draw up some Adrenalin' and 'start chest compressions' were passed around and we danced around one another like a well-rehearsed waltz, each taking on a task, all understanding that these next few minutes would mean the difference between life and death.

These moments are often over as quickly as they have begun, but it's always the unexpected ones that get to you. The young animals who have a whole life ahead of them. The preventable injuries and inexplicable drug reactions. We warn owners before every procedure that there is a risk of death with anaesthesia. But the truth is modern anaesthesia is very safe and many of the routine surgeries we carry out are on healthy young animals, lowering the risks even further. In a large study investigating small animal anaesthetic fatalities published in 2008, the overall risk of death with anaesthesia in dogs was found to be 0.17%, reducing to 0.05% in healthy dogs and rising only to 1.33% in sick dogs. So when the worst-case scenario actually happens, it is always a bit of a shock, no matter how many times you have experienced it.

Sarah made the call to stop attempting resuscitation ten minutes after chest compressions had begun and the room fell silent. Teddy had gone. As Sarah closed the surgical wound, I phoned the owner and tried my best to explain that due to events outside of our control, Teddy had not made it through his surgery. Their beloved, bright, bouncy, cheeky puppy would not be coming home to them. No, he didn't suffer, and yes, they could come in and see the body and say goodbye.

Later that evening, Sarah, Lucy and I sat side by side in the corridor outside theatre, tears in our eyes, dissecting what had happened. We hypothesised endlessly what had gone wrong, the 'could we have prevented it?' question weighing each of us down like a lead gown. In reality, we would never know exactly what had happened. Teddy had been suffering with an excruciatingly painful fracture, he was as cardiovascularly stable as possible prior to his surgery, and if we were presented with the case again, we would still make the same decision to operate a hundred times over. We suspected that he may have developed an embolus (travelling blood clot) related to his injuries, which had lodged in a lung or major vessel during the procedure, but whatever the cause it was outside of our control. Despite this, we each carried with us the heavy burden of guilt and sadness that descends upon every vet after an anaesthetic death.

We didn't make it out for a drink that night. The mood for partying had passed.

Part 2

WINTER

Christmas is always an interesting time for vets. It is generally known as the holiday season, but for those working in the veterinary profession, it is business as usual. Or more often than not, business multiplied by a few cases of mince pie ingestion, a handful of turkey bones lodged in dogs' intestines, the devouring of several boxes of Roses and Celebrations (with wrappers) and the classic string of tinsel lining a cat's intestines. For anyone not in the know, mince pies are toxic to dogs, as are many of the other consumables that might be lying around on the kitchen table during the festive period, such as grapes, onions, chocolate and alcohol.

Today's delight was Buddy, the six-month-old Leonberger puppy who had consumed an entire bottle of advocaat. He bounded in full of energy dragging his poor worried owner down the corridor and bashing into anything in his way, human or animal. He was on a drunken high much like a gaggle of tipsy vet students on a 2-for-1 cocktail night at the local student bar. After discussing the more serious side of things with his owner (alcohol is unfortunately highly toxic to dogs and can cause seizures, loss of consciousness, heart arrhythmias and, at worst, death), and establishing that this was an accident and wouldn't be happening again, we admitted Buddy for essential fluids and some quiet time in the hospital to consider his bad behaviour. His excitement soon turned to depression but luckily his blood tests were clear and he began to recover. I left him whimpering in his sleep this evening – it's going to be one hell of a hangover.

5 DECEMBER 2014

I have just finished looking at a urine sample under the microscope from a Staffie with kidney disease and a possible urinary tract infection (UTI). The owner, Mr Bailey, collected the sample from his dog at home as requested and dropped it in first thing this morning. I saw quite a lot of sperm in there – standard for an unneutered male dog. I then realised that the patient is castrated. There is zero possibility that a castrated male dog can produce sperm. This led me to the conclusion that it is, in fact, contamination from the handling of the sample. In other words, it's human sperm. I now feel a little queasy.

8 DECEMBER 2014

I heard some commotion in reception at the end of my shift today and ran down the corridor to see what was going on. I found James there with his friend Martin in hysterics with my favourite receptionist Emily. They had come to collect me after work to go to a carol concert that evening and Martin had thought it a great idea to come running into reception shouting that he had an emergency with his ginger ferret. I should point out now that James is a redhead and there was no actual ferret. Luckily, Emily, who is also part of the 'strawberry blonde' clan, is completely unflappable and has a good sense of humour. She realised very quickly that she did not need to run and grab a vet for the 'ferret emergency' because the 'ferret' was, in fact, my ridiculous husband. I apologised to her nonetheless and breathed a sigh of relief that there were no other clients (or ginger ferrets) sitting in reception.

10 DECEMBER 2014

I was reading up about a case today when Sally, one of the nurses, popped her head round the door and asked me to come quickly as there was an emergency. I walked into the clinic to find two young men standing next to their two-year-old black and tan Staffie, Ruby. Poor Ruby was lying on her side motionless. Her spine and ribs were very prominent and her eyes were sunken into her skull. The bones on her head protruded forward where normally thick muscle would be present. Her mammary glands were pendulous and bulky. As I approached I could see that they were red and engorged and one of them had formed an abscess which had ruptured, leaving a large open and oozing wound resembling the top of an active volcano. It was a fairly devastating scene. I examined her. She was alive, but barely. Her pulse was rapid and she had a high fever. She wouldn't last much longer without medical attention.

Sally and I rushed her through to our emergency room and placed a catheter in her flattened tiny vein, which is no easy feat in such a sick dog. I administered opioid pain relief and started her on what we call a 'shock dose' of fluids to help resuscitate her. We took blood samples, which Sally went to process while I walked back to the clinic room to talk to the owners. I needed to try and find out how on earth Ruby had ended up in this condition. While I had been gone Emily, the receptionist on duty, had checked eligibility and registered the client, whose name was Mr Kirwan. He was here with his cousin who helped him to 'care' for Ruby.

'Mr Kirwan, how long ago did Ruby have puppies?' I asked.

'Oh, around six weeks ago. But I've given them all away now.'

I decided to ignore the fact that the puppies were far too young to be taken away from their mother at this stage as I needed to concentrate on Ruby.

'How long has she been sick? She is in a terrible condition, Mr Kirwan.'

'Only a couple of days, yeah cuz?' He directed this question towards his sidekick for support. His cousin looked down at his feet, avoiding eye contact, and mumbled a monosyllabic 'yeah'.

I waited for Mr Kirwan to elaborate and after several moments he continued, 'She was fine, eating and stuff. She's always really hungry after her litters. It's her third one. The other times she's just bounced back. They kept feeding and feeding off her. There were eight of them. And then she got tired and just wanted to sleep all the time. She stopped eating a few days ago.'

'Did you increase her food intake after she gave birth to compensate for the milk she was producing?'

'Erm . . . she had her usual food. But she ate the puppies' food too when they had some.'

'Mr Kirwan, Ruby is extremely sick and could die from her condition. She should have been seen by a vet several days, if not weeks ago. Why were you unable to bring her in sooner?'

'I've been busy. And she seemed fine, she was just sleepy.'

'She was most likely sleepy because she is very poorly,' I said. Was he being naive or did he just not care? It was hard to tell.

'We will try everything we can to save her but you have a duty of care to your pets and leaving her to reach this state is not acceptable.' My tone was curt and frosty and an uncomfortable silence followed.

I prepared the paperwork and discussed a few further details before sending the client on his way. Before he left I asked, more out of my own curiosity, 'How much are you selling the puppies for?'

'Five hundred pounds a pup.'

Quite a profitable little business he has there.

I rushed back to Ruby. She appeared slightly stronger from the fluids and managed to lift her head as I entered the room. Her eyes were haunting, her expression one of a sullen acceptance that this was her fate. I rechecked her colour and pulse and then had another look at her mammary glands. The teats were raw and fetid brown material oozed out of them. They were swollen to the point of bursting and resembled the udders of a 500kg dairy cow prior to milking. This was the worst case of mastitis (infected breast tissue) I had ever seen and one of the worst neglect cases I had come across, on a par with Winnie. I started her on some intravenous antibiotics and we moved her carefully up to our dog kennels to settle her. It was going to be a long road to recovery for this little lady, involving weeks of anaesthetics to repeatedly flush and clean her wounds, and months of nutritional support. I wandered off sadly to go and talk to Esther who I knew would agree with me that this was a case for the RSPCA.

11 DECEMBER 2014

Today Eleanor the RSPCA welfare officer came to visit Ruby. Luckily she had improved significantly overnight and although she was still a very sick girl, she was out of the critically ill category. When I arrived at the hospital first thing this morning, she was ravenously hungry and eating everything in sight. She gulped her breakfast down like she'd never eaten before. It made me sad watching her. She was literally starving, her body having been stripped of each ounce of fat and every nutrient by a combination of eight hungry puppies feeding from her, lack of adequate nutrition and illness.

Eleanor took a statement from me. I hadn't quite understood how it worked before I graduated. The fact that vets don't have any legal rights to take an animal away from a home in which we believe they are being abused. Our first port of call in these scenarios is always the RSPCA officers who are legally trained and have the power to seize animals they believe are vulnerable or suffering. Eleanor took photos of Ruby from every angle to use as evidence. Even in the pictures you could see she was skin and bone. From above it looked like someone had crushed her into a 2D shape, flat Stanley style.

Eleanor decided after visiting the owner this morning and then assessing Ruby that she should be officially seized into RSPCA care. This meant that, until the court case at least, she would not be returned to Mr Kirwan and he would not be permitted any access to or given any information about her. She would stay in our care until she was medically well enough and then be kept safe in RSPCA kennels or a foster home until after the court case. If the judge decided she should not be returned to Mr Kirwan, which hopefully would be the case, then the search for her new family would begin. I felt a rush of relief. It was early days but her personality was already starting to shine through. She wagged her tail as I tickled her ears and sat obediently waiting for her bowl of food despite her savage and insatiable hunger. She let us prod and poke her and fiddle with her mastitis dressings without so much as a whimper. She was a patient and gentle soul.

'Don't worry, my friend. Things are going to improve for you from here on,' I whispered to her as I gave her a little cuddle.

12 DECEMBER 2014

Just seen a three-month-old puppy called Doodle for her first vaccinations. She was a delightful fluff ball with black and tan splodges, a white tummy and paws, floppy ears, a long shaggy tail, short stubby legs and a cheeky personality. I asked her owner, Mrs Wilson, how long she had owned her.

'Oh about ten days. Got her from this breeder I found online,' she told me. 'Paid eight hundred and fifty pounds for her, but she's a pedigree. A Yorkshire Terrier crossed with a poodle and a Shih Tzu.'

So she paid £850 for Yorkshire poo-shit. Otherwise known as a mongrel.

15 DECEMBER 2014

I saw a homeless man on our mobile van today, Mr Edwards with his ten-year-old Staffie, Jill. He's a lovely gentle man who absolutely adores his dog. As for many of our 'no fixed abode' (NFA) clients, she is his world. Unfortunately, and sadly, Jill has a large lump on one of her teats which I suspect is likely to be breast cancer. We discussed the options for treatment, including surgery and scans to assess for cancer spread, or referral to a cancer specialist which for Mr Edwards, as for many of our clients, would be prohibitively expensive. We then went through the aftercare and the necessity for shelter and a warm hygienic place for Jill to rest while she recovers. We would be able to keep her in the hospital for the initial few days after surgery, but after that he would need to find somewhere to stay with her.

It is three degrees outside today, and Mr Edwards had waited in the long queue of clients for nearly two hours to see me. He explained that he had been sleeping in a cardboard box for the last few months and had been homeless on and off for the last five years. During that time he'd had plenty of opportunity to take sheltered accommodation on the condition that he gave up his dog. They could not provide anywhere warm for him to sleep with Jill and he was not willing under any circumstances to part with her. This is sadly a relatively frequent situation for our NFA clients. He told me there was little else in his life that provided him with comfort, or a sense of 'family'. My heart suddenly ached for him as I listened to his story. It represented the ultimate bond between a man and his dog. He would rather risk freezing and starving to death than to be parted from her. His stomach must constantly cramp in desperate need of a hot meal and his bones must ache for a warm bed on these freezing British winter nights, but he would no more leave Jill out in the cold alone than anyone would leave their own child.

Sometimes I wish that people who don't have pets and don't understand their importance or why, as a society, we place so much emphasis on looking after them and educating people about their care, could step into my job for a day. Pets are a lifeline to a great number of people. Their welfare matters. Animals matter. Recent findings released by the family history website ancestry.co.uk indicated that more than a third of UK pet owners felt their pet was more beneficial to their life than humans, with 90% describing their pet as being part of the family. I quite agree. Some British pet owners even listed their dogs as 'sons' on the official forms of the 2011 Census. In a fast-paced world in which social media has caused us to question every facet of our being, animals teach us acceptance. They bring people together and transcend class, financial and cultural barriers. They are our loyal, loving, non-judgmental friends who allow us to just be ourselves, no questions asked.

There is a reason why dogs and horses have been used for many years as a form of therapy for humans to treat mental health disorders and to improve sensory issues among children with autism. The British Armed Forces use specially trained assistance dogs to help veterans suffering from PTSD. Schools have even started to promote a 'read to dogs' campaign following reports that children who read to pet dogs learn more quickly than those who read aloud to adults. Dogs will not judge them or laugh at their mistakes. Their mere presence creates a calming environment and encourages social interaction. And it's not just dogs who assist humans in this way. A study of over 600 people in the UK carried out by the Mental Health Foundation in conjunction with Cats Protection in 2011 also found that 87% of cat owners believed their pet improved their general well-being, while 76% said they could cope with everyday life much better in their presence.

Animals make us feel hopeful on the dark cold days and Jill was a prime example of this. There was a sparkle in Mr Edwards's eyes when he was talking to Jill. She lifted him from the emptiness of his reality and allowed him to maintain a sense of optimism and positivity. His bond with her was profound and her well-being was his upmost priority. She gave his life meaning and purpose. Typically for a Staffie, she was a soppy thing. Full of those wet sloppy kisses that happen so fast you only realise a tongue has crept into your nostril when you become aware of the warm gooey sensation spreading across your face. She lay on her back wagging her tail, desperate for tummy tickles. But one word uttered from Mr Edwards asking her to sit and she immediately obeyed. She gave me her paw as I offered her treats, and I snuck a few extra ones into Mr Edwards's hand as he was leaving. The date for surgery was set, but the question of aftercare still hung precariously in the air. She trotted out after him like his shadow, eyes fixed on him, and I wondered in the brief moment I had to myself before the next client stepped on to the van how he would cope when the time came for her to leave his side for ever.*

18 DECEMBER 2014

I have been given a mug for Christmas that says: *Please do not confuse your google search with my veterinary degree.*

Thank you, Santa.

Although God bless Google every time a bird, fish or any kind of amphibian or reptile walks through the door.

19 DECEMBER 2014

Received an email today from the hospital manager explaining that we currently have no money left in the company budget for stationery. I get that we have to pay for our own Christmas parties. We are a charity after all, and the yearly £10-a-head Christmas karaoke and cheap headache-inducing wine in the pub opposite the hospital has become somewhat of a tradition. But I'm not sure how I am going to explain to clients that we have no pens left and they are going to have to sign their pets' consent form with my liquid eyeliner.

22 DECEMBER 2014

I met my friend Mark for lunch today. It's always a bit of a gamble making lunch plans as Sod's Law dictates that it is inevitably the day multiple emergencies tumble in just as I am hoping to escape.

---

*Thankfully, in 2016 an RCVS-registered charity called Street Vet was created which delivers free treatment and preventative health care to the pets belonging to homeless people. The vets and nurses working for them are all volunteers out on the streets, pounding the pavements come rain or shine. They may not have been able to provide shelter for Jill but they could have picked up her cancer earlier, improving her chances of survival and reducing her post-op complication risk.

In fact, the last time I had made lunch plans with Mark on a work day, I had to get a colleague to call him to cancel as I was busy removing three litres of blood from a 50kg Rottweiler's chest. Luckily, today I managed to jump ship for forty-five minutes and see him. I arrived only fifteen minutes late to find Mark waiting patiently at our nearby sandwich shop. He is a mechanical engineer and works just down the road from me. Much like Chandler from *Friends*, I have never fully understood what his job actually entails. Something to do with computers and ventilation. I think.

'So, what have you been up to today?' I asked as we shared a mince pie.

'Oh, you know, winding down for Christmas,' he replied. 'My colleagues were ordering pizza as I left the office and we'll probably watch movies this afternoon.'

Words no vet has uttered, ever. Is this what normal people in normal jobs in normal offices do at Christmas time?

'How about you?' he asked.

On this particular morning, I had seen six itchy Staffies followed by Edgar the Bulldog who had eaten his big brother's epilepsy medication. His big brother is a 50kg Bull Mastiff and Edgar is a 2.5kg two-month-old puppy and he had arrived semi-comatosed. Thankfully he was looking much perkier by lunchtime after a bit of induced vomiting and a few hours on a drip. Edgar was followed swiftly by Suzie the tortoiseshell cat that had had seven seizures after her owner had applied a flea treatment meant for dogs over 20kg; she weighed 3kg and was evidently not a dog. Next was Bella the Staffie with a pyometra (infection of the womb) who had pus and blood oozing from her back end.[*] In the midst of the chaos I then sedated Princess the Chihuahua to numb her bad attitude and allow

---

[*]Womb infections are commonly seen in charity practice in unneutered female dogs. If left untreated, dogs with the condition ultimately die from septicaemia and the only successful treatment is surgery to remove the whole womb. It is one of the many reasons vets are so keen on neutering female dogs.

me to remove her ripped and haemorrhaging dewclaw. By the end of the morning there was blood and calamity everywhere.

I turned to Mark, considering how to answer his question. 'Oh, similar. Pizza and movies.'

23 DECEMBER 2014

Saw a lady today whose Jack Russell Terrier, ironically named Casanova, had paraphimosis. This means his penis was stuck out and he was unable to retract it back into its sheath. In Casanova's case it was most likely caused by excessive humping of his teddy bears at home. It can become a medical emergency if left untreated as the poor penis becomes swollen and engorged, which is pretty much as painful as it sounds. It was the third time I had seen Casanova for this condition in the last few weeks. I suggested that she gets Casanova castrated and in the meantime buys some KY jelly from the pharmacy to pop his penis back into its sheath herself, as time is of the essence when this condition occurs. She replied that she thought I was a pervert. In the age of Operation Yewtree I resented this accusation, but I smiled sweetly and directed her to the nearest pharmacy.

24 DECEMBER 2014

Everyone in the hospital was in a great mood today. One of the nurses spent the entire day wearing flashing reindeer antlers, there was a little plastic Christmas tree in reception and some wonderfully tacky tinsel lining the corridors. As a charity vet I have long since stopped dreaming of any kind of financial bonus at this time of year so you have to take joy in the small things. Plus I was working in theatre with two of my favourite nurses, Sally and Frieda, which was an extra Christmas treat. Both Sally and Frieda have been employed by PWH for nearly twenty years. They are very good nurses, but more importantly they are just lovely, kind people which makes all the difference in this job. The clients all seemed jolly despite their pets' various ailments, and to top the day off I ended up with a Chihuahua caesarean. Although it is not ideal being presented with a tiny dog that has been 'accidentally' mated with a Jack Russell Terrier twice her size, I still love a caesarean with a happy ending. The puppies were just so cute! People think that this job is mainly about playing with puppies and kittens all day. Well, today it was! I have named the two puppies (that's all she had room for in that tiny womb) Holly and Ivy. I'm sure the owner will rename them when they get home, but for now they have enforced Christmas names and that, along with the mulled wine I have consumed since the end of my shift, is making me exceedingly happy. Merry Christmas, furry friends.

28 DECEMBER 2014

Just finished a busy 24-hour on-call shift. The tube on the way home was completely dead despite being rush hour. Many people in Britain are tucked up with their loved ones, stuffing themselves with endless chocolates, bickering with family and exchanging gifts on these quiet precious days between Christmas and New Year. But not vets. Like the NHS, veterinary medicine never sleeps. The pre-Christmas cheer in the hospital has dulled and been replaced by a post-Christmas gloom. After a full day of consulting, I was thrown into an evening of blocked bladders, pyometras, a turkey bone stuck in an English Bulldog's intestine, a cat that had fallen from a fourth-storey window and shattered its pelvis (probably trying to escape the visiting relatives), a vomiting puppy and a kitten with diarrhoea, both of whom had been purchased, unsurprisingly, online.* And then, just when I lay my head on the

---

* A blocked bladder is just what it sounds like – a bladder that can't be emptied. This is a common feline emergency, often occurring in fat, stressed, indoor male cats belonging to multi-cat households. They become unable to pass urine and, if left, will die quickly and painfully.

pillow, a sixteen-year-old Collie called Sam was brought in at 4.30 a.m. He wasn't acutely unwell, but he had end-stage arthritis and Mrs Jackson had decided, after weeks of deliberating it and after spending 'one last Christmas together', to bring him in to have him put to sleep. I could have turned her away. Technically I don't need to see any non-life-threatening cases during emergency hours, but I just didn't have it in me. It had clearly taken a great deal of courage for Mrs Jackson to bring Sam in so I mustered my last iota of energy, compressed my frustration back into its box, and got on with the job.

I can still feel the adrenaline pumping through me several hours after the end of my shift. It's certainly much easier now, many years into the job than it once was. But I still find myself texting the vet whom I handed over to asking how my cases are doing or calling to remind the reception team that Mrs Bennet is hard of hearing and Ms Patel still needs to show her benefit details. As I sit stroking Bea and sipping a cup of tea trying to relax and wind down, I can't help reflecting on my first few emergency shifts as a new graduate. I had been warned by my university to try and find a supportive and nurturing first job that would help build my confidence and skill set as a newly qualified vet. PWH was everything I had wanted it to be and more in terms of opportunity to gain clinical expertise and experience a high turnover of new and interesting cases. But what it wasn't was a slow-paced calm environment conducive to gradual and supported learning. It was a 'throw you in at the deep end with bricks tied to your feet' sort of place. Sink or swim. There simply wasn't the time to mollycoddle new graduates. I had asked my first boss prior to taking the job what support I might receive out of hours, and her reply was very clear: 'In my day, we just got on with it.' This is an expression which has stayed with me, and one that many vets have sadly come up against at least once in their career. The 'we had it tough so you should too' school of thought, which takes no consideration of the mental health or easily shattered confidence of a new graduate. 'Oh, of course, well, I look forward to getting stuck in then,' I had replied, masking the terror I was feeling at the thought of sole charge of a five-tiered hospital with up to thirty inpatients at any one time and no previous experience of emergency work.

It's a curious thing, graduating as a vet. The day before graduation, you have your hand held throughout every consultation, every blood sample, every surgery if you are lucky enough to do any. And then you graduate after five years of training under experienced professors and clinicians, not seven years as is commonly believed, though it feels more like ten, and suddenly you are entirely responsible for every animal under your care. There is no compulsory postgraduate scheme or structured career ladder like in medicine, it's just a quick wave goodbye to your classmates and professors, a rather dry and lengthy graduation ceremony, and then off you go. You become a surgeon, medic and dentist to multiple species overnight. Fortunately, once I had started the job, I soon realised that the vets and nurses I worked with on the 'shop floor' at PWH were a lovely, supportive group who welcomed me into their dysfunctional yet endearing family with open arms. Within the first two weeks I had been handed backup phone numbers from Sarah, Lola and Lucy, like a toddler having a tantrum being handed pacifying candy.

'I have no plans this weekend, honestly, call me anytime if you need advice or support,' Sarah had said the day before my first night shift. Hearing those words made me feel immeasurably better. Even if I didn't end up calling her, just knowing that I could if I needed to was enough. My first few on-call shifts came and went rather uneventfully, with only a couple of minor inpatient incidents in the night.

'This isn't so bad, I can do this,' I thought to myself. Perhaps my fears of sole charge had been unjustified? About six weeks into my new job, however, I experienced a very different kind of on-call shift. The day on minors had been busy with a relentless stream of sick and difficult cases. My head was swimming with diagnoses and blood results, lists of owners I needed to call, and medications I needed to add to inpatients' kennel charts. By the time all my colleagues left at the end of the day I had several clinic appointments still waiting to be seen, including a possible blocked bladder and tortoise with a swollen eye, three transfers from other branches to admit to the hospital, plus a collapsed dog on his way down. I ran to the loo, which I had been postponing for several hours and found myself suddenly alone for the first time since my shift had started ten hours earlier. I was riding the wave of the on-call adrenaline high and felt a confusing mixture of complete control and utter panic about what was yet to come. Would I be able to handle it? Would my surgical skills be adequate? What if a more experienced surgeon could do a better job than me? What if I messed up or didn't know what to do? Too late for all that now. I pushed the niggling fears out of my head, gobbled down some congealed Percy Pigs from my locker for a much-needed energy boost, and rushed back to clinic to see the next client.

Later that night I admitted a Staffie that had been sent down to the hospital following an RSPCA visit after a neighbour reported seeing her lying lifeless on the balcony next door. Her name was Zia and she was a two-year-old sweet and gentle skinny little girl with a dark-brown coat and a white patch around one eye. She arrived extremely weak and pale with her tail tucked up between her legs and her head bowed low. She was white as a sheet and her heart was pounding. Her owner, Mr Vagueiro, was a tricky man to extract information from and each question I asked him was met with a monosyllabic response. There was a language barrier, but more significantly there was a distinct lack of trust on his part and I could tell that he would become aggressive if I probed further. I was very concerned about Zia and Mr Vagueiro agreed begrudgingly for us to admit her immediately to investigate her condition. I ran some blood tests and scans and took samples from her abdomen. She was bleeding internally. Oh no. Despite having been a vet for less than six months by then, I found myself rushing into theatre a short while later, aware that I would have to deal surgically with whatever I discovered in Zia's abdomen alone. I texted Sarah just beforehand for moral support.

'You can do this. Let me know how you get on!' she replied.

Deep breaths.

I clipped the fur around Zia's tummy when she was under anaesthetic and discovered several bruises that looked like they could be footprints. Just before midnight I started operating. As soon as I opened her up, blood gushed out of her abdomen. Soon enough there seemed to be blood everywhere. I couldn't suction it out fast enough. I desperately tried to pack her with swabs to stop the bleeding. I needed an assistant and an experienced surgeon with me. I tried not to panic. I was the best chance she had right now – the only chance she had – and I had to stay focused and calm. I had performed plenty of spays when I was abroad at the charity spay clinic over the summer and I knew I needed to apply the same gentle tissue handling skills I had learned during my training.

I soon found the source of the problem. Her spleen was twisted and had torn, causing major bleeding. It needed to be removed. I started to perform the procedure, but all of the familiar anatomy was obliterated by trauma and obscured by blood. I worked methodically along, all the while watching her blood pressure drop and her vital signs weaken. She needed a blood transfusion but we were a charity not a referral practice and we didn't have the time or resources to provide one. I couldn't help but think how different this situation would be if it were a person I was operating on in a human hospital. I took a deep breath and painstakingly continued to dissect each vessel that was attached to the bleeding spleen and tied it off. It was laborious work and I could feel sweat running down my back as I stood under the harsh glare of the theatre lights. My heart was pounding as I glanced at Sally, the nurse who was monitoring her anaesthetic, and saw the worried look on her face. 'Come on, work faster,' I told myself, and I noticed that my hands were trembling.

I finally finished the surgery, did my swab count, and closed Zia's abdomen as quickly as I could. I glanced at the clock. It was 3 a.m. and I hadn't stopped for more than five minutes in eighteen hours. My mind was frazzled. I went to the vets' flat once Zia was safely in recovery and collapsed on the unmade bed with the lights on, fully clothed. My heart was still pounding but I could feel the adrenaline crash coming as I stared in zombie fashion at the bright ceiling light above me. I must have drifted off because the next thing I remember was the loud and unforgiving sound of the vet phone ringing next to me. It was 5.08 a.m. I answered it and heard Sally's voice on the other end.

'I'm so sorry but I went to check on the blocked bladder cat and came back to find that Zia has passed away,' she said quietly.

Devastated doesn't quite cover the emotion I felt at that moment. I thanked Sally for letting me know and hung up the phone. And then it came. Great waves of emotion. Deep throaty sobs. That poor, young, unfortunate dog. What creature deserves to live and die like that? I felt anger towards Mr Vagueiro that I didn't know I possessed. I knew I had done everything I could to save her. And I knew that my bone-aching exhaustion and the chaos of the shift that came before it were exacerbating my feelings of crushing shock and grief for this little dog whom I had only met hours earlier. But I simply couldn't shake the sense that I had failed her somehow and I was haunted by the sad expression on her face as I had led her into theatre.

In the days and months that followed, my colleagues and university friends that I confided in about Zia told me repeatedly that I did everything expected of me and more and reminded me that often we see animals who are so sick that nothing we can do will fix them. My line manager at work was very supportive and I knew that the RSPCA would be taking matters into their own hands with regards to Mr Vagueiro. There would be an investigation and a court case and hopefully a fitting punishment. But I also knew that the memory of Zia and what had happened so early on in my new career would stay with me and would help to shape the vet I would become. My confidence and my heart had been dented, but I had also proved to myself that I could cope.

Sarah always describes these sorts of night shifts as 'character-building' and she is probably right. Since that night I must have done dozens if not hundreds more busy and overwhelming shifts like that. That's quite some character I must have developed by now.

In the years since I graduated, many veterinary practices including the charities have now started to offer new graduate internships in recognition of the additional support many newly qualified vets require at the start of their careers. These internships provide new vets with the opportunity to work in practice for lower salaries under the close guidance of a mentor, only doing emergency work when they feel ready and able to do so. It all seems a bit over the top to me – in my day, we just got on with it . . .

30 DECEMBER 2014

Me: . . . so the results have sadly come back and confirmed that Lilly has a type of cancer on her face.

Miss Hammond: But you have hacked her hair off! What about her television career? [Miss Hammond points to her Miniature Schnauzer's hair where it has been neatly trimmed prior to the biopsy of Lilly's cheek.]

Me: Yes . . . I can see that must be distressing for you. We had to cut a little bit of fur to make the procedure sterile and prevent infection, but it will regrow. Back to the results: we can consider referring her, but unfortunately there isn't anything we can do for her at our charity practice. The tumour on her face is inoperable.

Miss Hammond: OK. But she won't get called for any more auditions with this haircut. We were at a television studio last week for a special Christmas show and they won't want her back again. It's been completely hacked off. She's a television star you know!

Me: Aw, that's lovely. Good for her. And fingers crossed she will be able to go back for a short period of time once the hair regrows. But, Miss Hammond, do you understand what I'm saying to you about her cancer?

Miss Hammond: Yes. That it's bad and we can't do anything about it. I get it. As long as it doesn't affect her hair we can deal with it. It was so beautiful before, you know. She won't need chemo, will she? Then all her hair will fall out! But also the other thing I wanted to mention is that you didn't clip her nails when she was under the anaesthetic and I specifically asked you to . . .

Me: [Spontaneously combusts.]

5 JANUARY 2015

Today two unusual things occurred.

1. I got a pay rise. This never, ever happens. OK, well it wasn't exactly a pay rise, more just a 1% cost of living increase, but I'll take what I can get. Much to the surprise of most people, vets on the whole do not earn a lot. Our salaries are on average a third less than GPs and dentists and we certainly aren't 'in it for the money'.[*]
In fact, when I first graduated and was regularly doing 26-hour shifts, I once calculated that the additional hours supplement we received for these shifts worked out at less than £3 per hour.

2. I found a grass seed buried in a vagina. To be more specific, a Springer Spaniel's vagina. A grass seed! In January! Those little buggers get everywhere. It had looked so much like a nasty cancerous tumour, and the fact that I actually found it (it was a little like looking for a needle in a haystack) was a miracle in itself. For once I got to be the bearer of good news to an owner. The tumour was a grass seed!

Time for a glass of wine to celebrate.

[*]A study by the Department for Education and Institute for Fiscal Studies published in November 2018 revealed that veterinary medicine was in the bottom five jobs for earnings of female graduates in the UK.

8 JANUARY 2015

Saw Blaze last night, a one-year-old Boxer dog with a cough. His owner, a lady called Miss Page who I estimated to be in her forties but appeared initially older due to a mop of grey hair and several missing teeth, brought him in as an emergency. Blaze was a classic 'suspected non-emergency but can't be 100% sure as the owner is hysterical on the phone' case. So here he was at 2 a.m.

'Those pillow creases on your face are very endearing,' Miss Page's boyfriend remarked to me. I resisted the urge to raise an unimpressed eyebrow. I examined Blaze and sure enough he was fit as a fiddle, bar his hacking cough that I quickly ascertained was most likely caused by kennel cough (a highly contagious but usually non-life-threatening infection of the airways). He would not require any medication, just some TLC and to be quarantined from other dogs for a few weeks. I was starting to feel slightly irritated by the whole situation, having been dragged out of bed in the middle of the night as an emergency to see a dog who was essentially healthier than I was. Miss Page interrupted my thought process.

'I'm sorry if I've wasted your time, doctor', she said. 'I lost my mum last year and two weeks later I lost my dad. A month after that I lost my little Sampson from a brain tumour. I haven't been able to look at a Collie again since. But it's made me so paranoid about Blaze. I'm a bit overprotective now. I felt suicidal after Sampson went, but Blaze gave me hope again. I couldn't have children so they are my babies. Losing animals is so much harder than losing humans because they are never ever unkind to you.' In just a few sentences she had summarised many of the sad events of her life and my mood immediately shifted. Getting out of bed at 2 a.m. suddenly seemed a small price to pay to provide her with peace of mind.

'Don't worry at all, Miss Page, that's what we are here for,' I replied. 'It's always best to get these things checked. Better to be safe than sorry. And I am terribly sorry to hear about your losses, what an awful year you must have had.'

Miss Page sighed and I could see tears prick her eyes as she bent over and cuddled Blaze. Her boyfriend slipped awkwardly out of the door mumbling something about popping out for a cigarette. After he left Miss Page turned to me and rolled her eyes.

'They're weak things, men. Best to stick with dogs. Boyfriends come and go, dogs are for life.'

11 JANUARY 2015

The first three clients of my on-call shift today must have inspired the creation of the face-to-palm emoji. First up was Mrs Allen-Gonzaga who came in with two twitching and jerking three-month-old kittens.

'I gave them each a worming tablet yesterday and since then they've been like this,' she said, pointing to the little balls of twitchy fluff.

They seemed reasonably bright under the circumstances, but stumbled around slightly drunk with no apparent control over their muscles. One of them had recurrently twitchy whiskers on one side of his face and a flicking ear on the other side, while the second kitten had muscle spasm in his thigh and kept shaking his leg as if he had an itch that needed scratching. They were reminiscent of the aftermath of a veterinary student night out. The owner handed me the packet of worming tablets she had used to treat them.

'Mrs Allen-Gonzaga, these tablets are meant for large breed dogs,' I said patiently, pointing to the photo of the Golden Retriever on the front of the packet. 'It can be very dangerous giving the incorrect worming or flea products to your pet, especially to little kittens like these.'

'Oh, I did wonder why the tablets were so large. I had to break them into so many pieces to get them to eat the whole tablet.'

Face-to-palm moment number one. I checked the back of the packet and sure enough it contained an ingredient called permethrin that many over-the-counter flea and worming products contain, but which is unfortunately highly toxic to cats and can cause seizures and death in this species. I admitted the kittens to the hospital quickly and tried to calm their symptoms with muscle-relaxing and anti-seizure drugs, but knowing full well there was a chance they could deteriorate despite our best care.

Next up was Mr O'Brien with Biscuit, his three-year-old female Staffie who had had intermittent seizures for the last six months. I saw him at his previous appointment six weeks ago when I had recommended that we consider starting anti-epileptic drugs. This had also been suggested by colleagues before me during the two preceding appointments. The owner could not afford referral to investigate the cause of the seizures, and their frequency and intensity were getting gradually worse. Mr O'Brien had decided to ignore our recommendations and seek alternative treatment with a homeopathic vet. Cue face-to-palm moment number two.

Biscuit arrived having had six fits in a row this morning with only ten minutes between each one. Clearly the water infused with a mere whiff of something with a name I couldn't pronounce had not done the trick. I admitted Biscuit hastily, administered some non-homeopathic drugs to try and break the cycle of potentially life-threatening seizures and did my best not to judge Mr O'Brien when he told me he would really prefer to continue the homeopathic treatment after Biscuit had recovered. When it comes to alternative treatments, I do try to be open minded within the constraints of my evidence-based medical training. There is certainly a place for therapies such as acupuncture and herbal remedies as an adjuvant to the standard medical options. And I am all for clients seeking a second opinion if they don't feel confident about the information or treatment options being presented to them, but homeopathy is in a whole different category. What I really wanted to say to Mr O'Brien at that moment was that in my humble opinion (and the opinions of most of the vets in the UK), homeopathy was likely to be ineffective at managing his dog's seizures. It has no scientific basis whatsoever, which is hardly surprising considering it contains no active substances. By all means he should continue to use it alongside conventional medication as it is unlikely to be harmful considering it is essentially just water. But as his dog could die from her fits, I would highly recommend proceeding with drugs that have an actual evidence base behind them and are the best chance of saving her life.

As adult humans, it is our right to educate ourselves and make informed decisions about the medication we take based on the information we have available. If we wish to opt out of modern medicine in favour of alternative options then the only person we may be helping or harming is ourselves. But making decisions on behalf of our pets, in a similar manner to our children, carries a weightier level of responsibility. Animals may have no voice to make a choice for themselves, but they surely have the same right to treatment prolonging life and improving quality of life as people do.

When the moment arose, though, I knew my views on homeopathy would fall on deaf ears so I expressed a lighter version of this as gently as I could to Mr O'Brien. It was not the right time to get into a debate about homeopathy and my greatest concern was stabilising Biscuit.

Several hours later, once the kittens were looking more relaxed and had eaten some food and Biscuit was stabilised on his injectable dose of anti-epileptics, I saw my third face-to-palm client of the day. This one was a horror. Sweet Pea was a five-year-old Border Terrier who had been accidentally mated by a cheeky and apparently horny Jack Russell in the park earlier this morning. Miss Kurtis, in her disgust at the situation and haste to separate them, had physically ripped them apart after they had locked on to one another.

For those that are unfamiliar with dog mating, dogs begin having intercourse like many other species. The female stands on all fours and the male jumps on her back, grips on to her and humps away – nothing unusual there. This process lasts about five minutes or so while they get comfortable together and during this period a gland at the head of the dog's penis, called the bulbus glandis, swells and enlarges, locking his penis inside the female's vagina. This is called the 'copulatory tie'. What is different about dogs is that the next step in the process involves the male dismounting from the female with his penis still inside her so that they are stuck in a back-to-back tie. They are literally locked together, and can stay this way for up to forty minutes until the bulbus glandis starts to shrink and they are able to separate. If they are physically separated before they are ready, a great deal of damage can be done to their internal organs.

'I think she's bleeding from the back end a bit,' Miss Kurtis said, looking remarkably calm and stoney faced. 'I had to really yank them apart,' she added.

Super.

I examined Sweet Pea, expecting some trauma but hoping for the best based on how underwhelmed the owner seemed about the situation. That was an error. I was met with a grizzly scene. Sweet Pea's entire vagina had been ripped apart. I could barely make out any of her external genital anatomy. I am not easily shocked but this was pretty horrendous. I was fairly certain I could see faeces from her bowel inside her vagina, and the whole area had swelled up into a large red balloon. I explained to the owner how grave the situation was and was met with a monosyllabic response. I couldn't work out whether she was feeling very guilty and was thus subdued, or whether she really just didn't care. I was hoping for the former but feared the latter.

I admitted Sweet Pea to hospital for emergency treatment. After administering some heavy-duty painkillers, I anaesthetised her to try and work out what on earth had happened. As I suspected, there was a complete laceration through her vagina into her bowel. I placed a catheter into her bladder to make sure she could urinate and started her on antibiotics. It was all looking very crusty by this point and the potential for infection was high.

I took photos of the disaster zone to discuss the case with my colleagues, placed a special dressing, and patched her up as best as I could, but she would need more specialist surgery the next day and would probably end up being in and out of the hospital for several weeks. I still wasn't sure if she'd make it.

I have seen a fair number of frustrating cases over my time in charity practice, including plenty of wounds caused by owners trying to separate fighting or mating dogs. One dog that stands out in my mind came in with burns across her entire back as the only way her owner could think of separating the dogs from fighting was to pour boiling water all over her. But Sweet Pea had to be up there with one of the worst cases of accidental owner-induced trauma I have seen. The force Miss Kurtis used to separate the dogs must have been considerable, even if her intentions had been good. Why not just get your dog neutered if you are that desperate to ensure they don't breed? With so many other health benefits, it seems like a no brainer to me. I checked the time on my phone. It was only midday. How was that possible?! Nine hours of my shift left to go. I sighed and opened a text from James asking how my day was going. I pinged him back several face-to-palm emojis and felt immediately better.

13 JANUARY 2015

First five appointments on today's day list:

'Pepi' Coughlan, eight-year-old Chihuahua – coughing.

'Peewee' Thomas, three-year-old cat – straining to urinate.

'Red' McDonald, five-year-old Rhodesian Ridgeback – feeling blue.

'Chubs' Boon, four-year-old Persian cat – off her food.

'Chewy' Holmes, two-year-old Siamese cat – chewed through a glow stick.

14 JANUARY 2015

I bumped into my neighbour Alex last night on my way home from work. He mentioned that he and his girlfriend were in the process of trying to adopt a new cat and had tried many rehoming centres but had so far been unsuccessful. He was now considering looking online, or at local adverts in magazines and was asking my advice about it.

I was surprised to hear that Alex wasn't able to find the cat he wanted from a rehoming centre as he lives in a nice house with a garden, on a quiet road and with no other pets. When I probed him about it, it transpired that the reason he was being turned down time and time again by the centres was because he wanted an unneutered female cat that he could breed from. He explained to me that he had always had cats since he was a young child and that they had always had a few litters of kittens each.

My neighbour is responsible and kind to his cats and they have always lived long and happy lives. His previous cat had passed away recently at the age of seventeen. He told me that both he and his girlfriend had done their homework about how to look after the mum cat while she is pregnant and lactating and how to look after the kittens after they are born. He added that in the past he had always found loving homes for all the offspring. So why wouldn't the rehoming centres give him an unneutered female cat? Why was he forced to purchase a cat privately online when he wanted to rescue an unwanted cat from a rescue charity?

Well, why indeed?

Aside from the fact that the majority of owners in the UK get their cats neutered and therefore many of the strays that end up at rehoming centres are already neutered, there is then the issue of feline reproduction. Cats are notoriously fertile creatures. Female cats enter puberty as early as four or five months old, which is why most animal charities recommend neutering at this age. Any time from then on they can get pregnant, and will be jumped on by any keen and willing tomcat lurking around the neighbourhood. In fact, female cats (or Queens as they are called) often mate with multiple toms over a number of days and the resultant litter may have several different fathers. They are just babies still at this age, with undeveloped growing bones unsuited to carrying a litter. It would be no different to a thirteen-year-old child getting pregnant, other than the fur and the fact they can carry as many as eight offspring per pregnancy. Feline pregnancies last just over two months, so let's say our hypothetical kitten has a litter when she is around eight months old. Cats are induced ovulators, which means they produce an egg each time they have sex and can be sexually active again in as little as two weeks after giving birth. So if we assume a minimum of two to three litters per year and up to eight kittens per litter, that one cat and its kittens could produce as many as 420,000 kittens in just seven years. People call neutering 'unnatural'. In the wild, yes, cats would mate and give birth regularly. But in the wild they would also die young from horrible painful infections, get into fights that would leave them with a permanent limp or the loss of vision in an eye, and spend their days hungry and riddled with parasites. This is surely not how we want our domesticated pets to live.

Aside from the risk of sexually transmitted diseases and the miserable existence that comes with being a continual breeding machine, I also hate to think what the UK would look like if we allowed our cats to reproduce in this way. Having spent many holidays abroad dragging James around the streets of Greek islands with packets of ham and foreign cat food, feeding the flea-ridden pregnant Queens and war-torn toms that live there as strays, I am so pleased we take animal welfare seriously in the UK. I have worked with two animal welfare charities in Southern Europe since I graduated and was dismayed by the conveyer belt of stray dogs and cats being brought in from the streets day after day to be neutered. These animals needed and deserved companionship, security, nutrition and, above all else, a loving home, but many of them would never experience the simple pleasures that we take for granted in Britain.

Unfortunately, though, despite our fantastic neutering rate in the UK and the subsidised neutering schemes offered by rescue organisations, we still have a fight on our hands. We may not have animals wandering around the streets like they do in Southern Europe and Asia, but our centres are all full to bursting with more and more cats being abandoned. Several charities have clubbed together under the umbrella of the Cat Population Control Group (CPCG) to reduce the number of unwanted cats being born in the UK. But still cats are being put to sleep every day in rehoming centres because we simply can't find homes for them all. I tried to explain this situation to Alex. Of course I wasn't suggesting for a moment that he would let his cat spend a lifetime producing kittens. But the rehoming centres don't know him and cannot predict which owners will breed responsibly and then get their cat neutered, and which will not. Once they leave the safety of our care, we have to be absolutely sure they are going to have as safe, happy and healthy a life as possible.

Today I was on our mobile van and the first two patients of the day were cats. Boots was a ten-year-old cat that hadn't eaten for a week and had pus pouring out of her back end. She was not neutered and I soon established that the pus was coming from her womb. She had a life-threatening pyometra. I sent her straight down to the main hospital to be stabilised for emergency surgery.

The second cat, Philippa, was a two-year-old cat that was pregnant with her fourth litter. She lived with two of her eight-month-old daughter cats, both of whom were also at risk of getting pregnant. Philippa was skinny and covered in fleas and had an infected wound on one of her legs. There was limited treatment I could give her in her impregnated state so I patched her up as best as I could and sent her on her way. Before the owner left I booked all three cats in to be spayed (Philippa once she had given birth to the latest litter), but I had a feeling that the owner would miss her appointments. I reflected momentarily on my chat with Alex the night before and felt reassured that our rehoming centres are standing strong and refusing to send unneutered cats out to new homes. How could we possibly justify it under these circumstances? I'm relieved to say that every cat that leaves the doors of a PWH rehoming centre has been neutered, microchipped, health checked by a vet and treated for parasites. In the case of older or unwell animals they may have even had investigations, dental work, medicine or surgery to improve their quality of life or treat conditions such as thyroid disease prior to being sent out to their new home. This is standard for the majority of dog and cat rehoming charities across Britain, and in my opinion it's absolutely how it should be.

16 JANUARY 2015

Today Mrs Briggs brought her cat Elsie to see me. Elsie is a six-year-old Tabby cat in robust health. Mrs Briggs, on the other hand, has Munchausen by proxy and brings all three of her cats in on a regular basis with a variety of suspected ailments.[*] The trick is to recognise the few occasions when they're actually unwell, which is not easy when the preceding twelve visits have amounted to nothing more than increasing her pets' stress levels. I do have sympathy for Mrs Briggs as I think part of the issue is that, in addition to her fragile mental health, she is lonely. We see cases like this commonly in the veterinary charity sector where we are dealing with vulnerable members of society. Mrs Briggs has little else going on in her life and her visits to see us are a dominant part of her weekly plans. By her own admission, she lives alone apart from her feline family and she 'doesn't care much for humans'. I wonder if the latter is true, or that perhaps it is sadly humans who haven't cared much for her over the years.

[*] Munchausen by proxy is a condition that usually affects adults caring for children but also applies to pets, whereby the carer fabricates or exaggerates health problems in those who are under their care. In this case, the dependants in question were Mrs Briggs's cats.

Each visit, Mrs Briggs brings a letter detailing her concerns, with dates and times of all relevant occurrences – coughs, wheezes, changes in appetite, faecal consistency and so on. She went through a phase, when one of her older chubby cats was on a prescription diet for obesity, of detailing each ingredient and the manufacturer's code for the food, and firing numbers at me every visit from behind her disconcertingly thick half-moon spectacles. I'm still not quite sure how she expected me to respond to her question, 'I ordered code number 36854 but number 36855 has three per cent more fat than the 27858 and contains pork and chicken liver compared to 58920 which has over six per cent fat. So should I order the 58920, the 27858 or the 36854?'

Eh? It was like some kind of elaborate riddle. Luckily, Herbert wouldn't eat any of the food we recommended, which brought a timely end to the problem. Herbert has since lost 2kg simply by reducing his normal portion of daily kippers.

Today's suspected ailment was 'gingivitis', aka sore gums. She had looked it all up on the Internet and had meticulously written notes about which days Elsie appeared to have had bad breath or chewed on the left side rather than her usual right side. She didn't even want her kippers for breakfast one day which was most unlike her. I examined Elsie and sure enough, in the words of Mary Poppins, her teeth were 'practically perfect in every way'.

'Mrs Briggs, I don't think we need to do anything about Elsie's teeth at the moment,' I said as gently as possible.

'But she's clearly got gingivitis. Here, look at this picture,' she replied, reaching for a photo she had printed from the Internet of a cat with gingivitis. 'They look the same! And her breath! She has to have a dental.'

'We don't perform anaesthetics lightly. They carry risks, albeit very small risks in a healthy cat, but I wouldn't want to do dental work on her unless it was really necessary.'

'I appreciate what you're saying, Charlotte' (oh God, she remembered my name), 'but she could end up with something far worse like an abscess of a molar tooth without it.' It's always unnerving when a non-medic casually throws clinical terms into the mix.

'She is highly unlikely to get an abscess when she has minimal tartar on her teeth and no evidence of the development of infection. We can monitor her regularly and if we become concerned we will let you know.' I stood my ground. My colleagues would not be impressed if I landed a dental on their list that didn't need doing, not to mention the fact that it would be morally wrong.

'You said "unlikely" but that means you can't be certain,' she went on, undeterred by what I thought had been my entirely convincing response.

'Medicine is rarely black and white, and few things are certain. But I can tell you from all my years of experience that I'd be completely shocked if she had any medical issues related to her teeth being dirty in the coming months. And in the meantime we can start her on a special dental care dry food to help her maintain good oral hygiene.'

'Oh, you mean number 38591 . . .'

Nooooooo!

19 JANUARY 2015

We had a seizuring dog in the hospital today that I struggled to stabilise. He was an old Boxer called Bruce and he came in looking slightly dazed and almost immediately collapsed to the floor having a full-blown fit. I have seen it so many times now that it no longer shocks me, although I find that the bigger the animal the more difficult it is initially to try and take control of the situation. He was thrashing around with his eyes rolled back, frothing at the mouth, legs splayed wildly and his whole body twitching uncontrollably. The owner was distraught. As I reached for the drugs I needed and the nurses and other veterinary colleagues rallied around me to place an intravenous catheter, check his temperature and vital signs and take blood samples, I was reminded of one of the first times I had been presented with a seizuring case as a new graduate.

It was my third week working at PWH and I was still learning the ropes. Historically, the relationship between vets and veterinary nurses hasn't always created a friendly or productive working environment, a phenomenon that is also well documented in human medicine. Indeed there has been, and still is, potential for animosity between the two working groups, with many veterinary nurses feeling communication with vets is unsatisfactory and that they are not always treated with the respect they deserve. The framework (and its limitations) that we all have to work within can heighten the potential for such tensions. Veterinary nurses are often caring for multiple patients at a time and cannot always carry out a vets' request for a patient immediately. Similarly, vets often walk around in a cloud of semi-confusion, with test results to interpret, owners to call and drug doses to alter and this can mean we don't always remember to complete simple tasks such as unblocking a patient's drip line when we walk past a beeping machine or shutting down our computer at the end of a clinic session. This can be incorrectly interpreted as laziness when in reality it is often due to an overburdened, frazzled mind that cannot accommodate any more jobs on an ever-expanding to-do list.

Having observed difficulties between vets and nurses in my university practice placements, I knew that as a newly qualified vet it would be important to form strong working relationships with the nurses looking after my patients. At the charity practice I had volunteered for in Lisbon after graduation, the vets worked alone with no nursing assistance, performing operations while simultaneously managing and monitoring the anaesthetics. It had been almost impossible and emphasised how lucky we are in the UK to work alongside well-trained veterinary nurses. I don't think I realised, however, just how integral they are to the normal functioning of the hospital, or how their knowledge and experience would be crucial to my first few weeks and months in practice.

When a Rottweiler arrived having a non-responsive seizure, I completely froze. The knowledge was all in my head from years of studying at university but I lacked the vital experience required to deal with the situation. I distinctly remember standing in our emergency room like a deer in headlights with the Rottweiler lying at my feet convulsing and a room full of people looking at me, waiting expectantly for me to take control of the situation. I knew I had to pull myself together or the dog would die.

'Do you want us to place an intravenous catheter?' Sophie suggested, already getting material prepared.

'Yes. Good idea,' I muttered, while flipping through my drug formulary trying to locate the right dose of the anti-epileptic drug I needed to give.

'Shall we take a blood sample at the same time?' Emma asked as she grabbed the syringe and blood tubes from the cupboard.

'Yes please,' I replied. I had managed to locate the page I needed and was furiously tapping numbers into a calculator.

'We have rectal diazepam available if that's any help?' Frieda mentioned from across the room.

'Yes! Great, let's get some of that on board,' I said.

And so it continued until the dog was eventually stabilised. The truth is that when you first graduate you don't have a clue how to manage emergencies or how to collate the information you have in your brain and transform it into real-life actions. Although I'm hugely grateful to all my veterinary colleagues for their support in my early years of training, I also owe a mammoth amount of gratitude to the nurses who held my hand and guided me through many a sticky moment.

Sadly, back to today, Bruce was too sick to stabilise fully. I suspected a brain tumour and he was put to sleep this afternoon surrounded by his sobbing family. I watched Frieda writing a condolence card to the owner and carefully attach the lock of hair inside the card that the owner had asked us for. She then dabbed his paw with ink and gently placed it on the condolence card to make a paw print keepsake for them. It takes a special kind of person to be a veterinary nurse. Despite having the knowledge and experience required to take control of a seizuring patient all these years later, I had still relied heavily on the nurses to deal with Bruce. I am proud to call many of the nurses I work with my friends as well as colleagues. I have learned that it is OK to have my medical decisions questioned or feedback given to me on aspects of patient care by other staff members. Kindness and mutual respect leads to an inclusive working environment and helps us all to cope with the pressures of the job. Vets cannot function alone. We need our nurse partners-in-crime and would be lost without them.

21 JANUARY 2015

I decided to start following Ricky Gervais on social media today. It seems an odd choice for me as I'm not usually much of a 'tweeter'. I only post occasionally and even then it's usually a photo of Bea's face from a slightly different angle to the one I posted six months before. I'm not generally prone to following actors or musicians online but he caught my eye through his use of social media to promote animal welfare. He has helped to raise awareness for the #adoptdontshop campaign, a slogan that a growing number of animal rights proponents have been using to encourage the adoption of pets from shelters rather than purchasing them from breeders or online. He also tweets links to petitions about freeing animals who are being treated poorly in captivity and has spoken out about fox hunting and bullfighting. It's funny how an interest and concern for animals can bond you to someone you've never met and probably have little else in common with. Keep up the good work, Ricky!

22 JANUARY 2015

I walked into the cat kennels this morning to find Sophie popping Diego on to a cat bed for the day, moving at the pace of a sloth and slightly hunched like a little old lady. As she turned around, I gasped. Her entire body was absolutely covered in puncture wounds and scratches. Her hands were swollen and her fingers resembled green sausages that had been stabbed by a skewer multiple times.

'Soph, what on earth happened!'

'Oh God. It was awful. I spent the last twenty-four hours in A&E on IV antibiotics.'

'But what actually happened to you? Are you OK? You look like you've been attacked by a lion!' I had visions of some wild beast that she'd taken into the New Hope charity attacking her in the dead of night.

'It was this little female kitten. I was transferring her in a cat carrier and she escaped! I ran after her and then somehow I managed to catch her. But then I realised that I had no protection, no towel, no gloves, no basket, just me and her lying on the ground with me clinging on as tightly as I could. I thought if I let go, I'd never see her again and she'd go off and have an awful life on the street and get pregnant or run over. So I just kept holding her. But she's a wild little beast so she resisted and started attacking me. She bit me and scratched and wiggled and yowled and all the time I just clung on and on until she eventually calmed down. Thank God my colleague at New Hope came and found us.'

'Oh my God, Soph, that's madness! You could have died from shock or sepsis with all those bites! For goodness' sake, you have to be careful and look after yourself!'

'I know, that's what they said at the hospital. I ache all over.'

Sophie lifted up her scrub trouser legs to reveal her swollen and bruised legs covered in bites. I had never seen anything like it. I imagined the horrified look on the doctor's face in A&E when she rocked up half dead with her story about saving a little feral cat.

Thank the Lord for antibiotics or she'd be a gonner for sure. It is astounding the lengths some of my colleagues will go to in order to protect animals, but Sophie always takes it one step further. She is one of the few people I know who is crazy enough to lay down her life for a wild terrified cat. That's one lucky feline, although I get the feeling she may not be the grateful type.

23 JANUARY 2015

I thought I was having a bad week. My boiler broke last night and it was snowing so I boiled kettles of water, made a tepid bath, and sat shivering and feeling sorry for myself. I didn't sleep well after that. My essays for my certificate were due in and I stayed up until late trying to finish them. Veterinary certificates are postgraduate qualifications that many vets undertake to gain expertise in a specific field while continuing to work as general practitioners. Within a few years of graduating I had enrolled on a certificate programme in small animal medicine. Basically, I got bored despite the complexity and fast pace of the job and wanted more letters after my name than my husband, and to continue down the route of stress, anxiety, essays and exams that I swore after graduating I would never do again. You have to have a particular type of personality to become a vet, aka self-confessed workaholic and masochist, aka idiot.

So I had woken up in a grump after five hours' sleep, left the house without washing due to aforementioned boiler issues, and then received a text from my friend saying our weekend plans had fallen through as she had norovirus. Terrific. I stomped through the melting slush to the tube station to work feeling very sorry for myself. My first client of the day, Mrs McCarroll, came in with her dog Scruff. Scruff was a very sweet, but slightly crusty ten-year-old Bichon Frise with large bulging eyes between which lay, I suspected, a rather small brain. Scruff had keratoconjunctivitis sicca (KCS), otherwise known as 'dry eye'. This is a relatively common chronic condition where the surface of the eye becomes irritated by a lack of tears. Part of the treatment involves placing artificial tear drops into the eyes regularly throughout the day.

Last time I had seen Mrs McCarroll, a lovely Irish lady in her mid seventies, she had been struggling with Scruff's eye medication because she was developing cataracts herself and was also the sole carer for her sick husband. That was about six months ago. As soon as Scruff entered the room my heart sank. The small part of his right eye that I could see was bright red, there was pus pouring from it and he was holding it firmly closed and was in considerable pain. The last entry on the medical history, written by me six months earlier, said: *Advised owner not to run out of meds, discussed long-term nature of condition and potential suffering and blindness if left untreated.*

I learned early on in my job to give people the benefit of the doubt. You see a lot of animal suffering in this profession, particularly in the charity sector. But you also see a lot of human suffering. By law every owner has a duty of care under Section 9 of the Animal Welfare Act to ensure they take reasonable steps to meet the welfare needs of their animals. If an animal's welfare is compromised, then an owner may receive a formal warning or even be prosecuted depending on the nature of the offence. But although there is a percentage of people who should not own animals as they are unable or unwilling to put the time or effort into their care, there is also a large percentage of people who don't mean to harm their pets. They love them and care for them to the best of their abilities, but due to disability or illness or other life events beyond their control, they are simply unable to fulfil their duty of care to the extent they should. These are the 'benign neglect' cases and are extremely difficult to deal with as no one is really to blame.

Working in charity practice alongside life's most poorly educated and least fortunate people, I have seen more than my fair share of welfare cases, and likely many more than my peers working in private practice. Within my first four years at PWH I had been involved in three RSPCA neglect cases that ended up in court, and I am only one of the twelve vets working in my hospital. This also doesn't include animals like Winnie where the owner is never prosecuted, or stray animals that are brought in by members of the public which have suffered at the hands of their owners who will never be found. That is a lot of animal abuse. As a result, I have rapidly become a good judge of whether intentional cruelty has occurred. In this particular instance, yes, an animal was suffering and veterinary treatment should have been sought sooner. But no, I don't believe Mrs McCarroll deliberately harmed her pet or intended for him to suffer.

I examined Scruff, who was extremely tolerant under the circumstances, and established that he had a deep infected melting ulcer and would need very intensive treatment to attempt to salvage the eye, otherwise enucleation (removing the eye) would most likely be on the cards.* I gently probed Mrs McCarroll about how he had reached this state and with very little prompting she began to explain that she simply cannot see his eyes any more, and only realised how bad they had become when her daughter came to visit. She hadn't managed to come back sooner because her son had died suddenly and unexpectedly following a procedure in hospital that had not gone to plan, and then her brother had also passed away. She was still the sole carer for her husband who had Alzheimer's disease and after fifty-two years of marriage he no longer recognised her and he had started to become physically aggressive towards her after being a gentle man all his life. I listened as she continued to tell me intimate details of her life in an entirely stoic and matter-of-fact manner, each event enough to place strain on the most stable person's mental health, and together enough to push most people into a hole of despair. Yet it was only when I mentioned that Scruff was in pain and might end up losing his eye that Mrs McCarroll finally cracked. The tears rolled down her cheeks and all the months of sadness seemed finally to hit her at the mention of her beloved pet being so unwell.

---

* A melting ulcer is an ocular emergency. It is essentially a large melting hole in the surface of the eye that is collapsing in on itself and can rapidly lead to rupture of the eye. In this case it was almost certainly caused or exacerbated by the underlying condition (KCS) being left untreated for so long.

She said very quietly in a trembling voice, 'He's all I've got now you see, my dear. Him and my daughter, but she has her own life. Scruff helps me get through each day.'

I suddenly felt very small and deeply sad for this lovely lady in front of me, and the cruel hand the universe had dealt her. My own boiler and weekend plan woes seemed pathetic in comparison.

'Don't worry. He's in good hands,' I reassured her. 'You've done exactly the right thing by bringing him here. We will do everything we can to help him.' And I squeezed her arm before she handed him over to me and backed away like a deflated balloon out of the door.

I went home at the end of my shift and hugged James and Bea tightly and only moaned a tiny bit about the boiler.

27 JANUARY 2015

Mr Santos and his Beagle Harry came into clinic today, having visited Dr Google before they arrived. A nationwide survey of vets by the BVA in 2014 revealed that 98% of vets feel their client's behaviour is influenced by what they find online, with only 6% of vets finding owners' online research helpful. Unsurprising. Unfortunately, Mr Santos fitted into the 'unhelpful' majority.

Me: What's up with little Harry today?

Mr Santos: I just need some antibiotics for his skin.

Me: Let's have a little look at him. Why do you think he needs antibiotics?

Mr Santos: I don't need a discussion, I've already been waiting an hour. I just need the medicine. He had it last time and I want it again.

Me: [Checks computer notes. Last time we gave anti-inflammatories for a sore foot.] I'll just have a look at Harry and then we can decide what treatment he needs.

Mr Santos: I read about it on Google. It's mange.[*]

Me: What makes you think it's mange? Has he had any recent parasite treatment? Is he itchy? Any other problems? Eating and drinking OK?

Mr Santos: I told you, I read about it on Google. No, he's fine. I told you it's his skin. If you don't give me the antibiotics then on your head be it. If he dies overnight it's your fault.

Me: [Assesses the patient, who is extremely bright and bouncy and trying to bite me, and has a very small area of red skin on his neck where his collar has been rubbing.] Mr Santos, I completely understand your concerns but this doesn't look like mange to me and antibiotics aren't the recommended treatment for mange anyway. I think you should purchase a harness as his collar is rather tight and rubbing against his neck. And I would highly recommend covering him monthly for parasites. We have a spot-on treatment you can buy from us here that also covers for fleas and lungworm.

Mr Santos: I told you, it's mange. If you can just give me the antibiotics then I will leave. I'm not paying for any poxy flea treatment. I'm on benefits!

Me: Mr Santos, I . . .

Mr Santos storms out of the clinic.

30 JANUARY 2015

Finally finished a busy day of consulting. My last appointment of the day was a mother in her eighties and daughter in her fifties

---

[*]Mange is a type of skin disease caused by parasites called mites. There are two main types of mange in dogs – sarcoptic mange (scabies) and demodectic mange, both of which can be safely and effectively treated by antiparasitic medications prescribed by a vet. Dr Google recommends using honey, olive oil or bathing in hydrogen peroxide. Don't believe everything you read . . .

with their sixteen-year-old cat Georgie for a 'newly diagnosed diabetic' consultation. This was meant to be booked as a double appointment with a vet to discuss the condition, followed by a double appointment with a nurse to demonstrate how to administer the insulin injections.* Unfortunately, it had been booked as a single appointment for a vet and I was informed politely but firmly by the clinic nurse that there were no nurses available for the nurse appointment due to staffing issues. I called the clients into my consultation room, aware of the fact they had already been waiting for over an hour and wondering how I would be able to fit forty minutes of information into ten.

It became clear to me almost immediately that this was not going to be a quick appointment. Thank goodness I had no plans tonight. Mrs Meldrow, the older lady and actual owner, was beside herself. Her husband had died last year and Georgie was his cat. She was the last thing Mrs Meldrow had left of him. This is a common story, one I hear most days at work, and yet it still gets me every time. Mrs Meldrow was soft and gentle in nature, her grey hair thinning and styled up into a bouffant with a large purple clip. She wore bright pink lipstick and despite the fact that her eyes were yellowing at the edges and surrounded by the creases of a lifetime, their light blue sparkled as she spoke animatedly about Freddy, the love of her life. They had been married for sixty-two years. Georgie would only ever sit with him. She didn't like anyone else and would hiss when visitors came to the house. She followed Freddy around like a shadow. Since he passed away, she had started to sit with Mrs Meldrow. Some days she felt that Freddy was trying to communicate with her via Georgie to let her know that everything was going to be OK.

Oddly, Mrs Meldrow's daughter, Ms Turner, had a very different vibe to her mother. She was cold and abrupt, mouth pouted and slightly turned downwards, and she avoided eye contact. She

---

*Diabetes Mellitus in cats is treated with daily insulin injections, similar to type 1 Diabetes in humans.

disagreed with her mother about small trivial pieces of information, such as what year Freddy had been diagnosed with cancer or how many times a day Georgie had been vomiting. When I asked questions about how they felt about treating Georgie, Mrs Meldrow replied that she wanted to do anything she could to save her. Ms Turner asked with a hint of aggression what she would do when she had theatre tickets and wanted to go out for the evening instead of going around to her mother's house to inject the cat. Oh dear. I gradually realised the issue. Mrs Meldrow's hands were gnarled and swollen and drawing up minute doses of insulin into a syringe every day was going to be an impossibility. Ms Turner was clearly underwhelmed at best by the prospect of visiting her mother every day at the same time of day to help her to inject Georgie.

I examined Georgie who was emaciated because of her condition but bright and comfortable enough. Being a medic, diabetes is one of the conditions I enjoy treating the most because there is so often something that can be done about it. But treatment is a huge commitment, and in private practice a huge expense, and not every client chooses to proceed with it. Some opt for euthanasia instead. I mentioned this option cautiously and gently to Mrs Meldrow, but it initiated a new flood of tears and a new wave of tutting and impatience from her daughter. I glanced at the clock. It was thirty minutes into the consultation already and forty minutes beyond my official end of shift time and I hadn't even shown Mrs Meldrow how to administer the injections yet. I glanced at the day list for the next day. It was fully booked. I knew Ms Turner would not want to come back again anyway. Georgie would eventually die without treatment, and Mrs Meldrow could not bear to consider letting her go – at least not today. Ms Turner was our only hope. I sighed inwardly, settled into my chair and picked up the box of syringes and needles and bottle of sterile water for injection practice and began my explanation.

3 FEBRUARY 2015

Saw a lovely client called Mr Michael today, a man in his sixties with his new German Shepherd puppy named Martha. She was absolutely gorgeous, all soft and fluffy and edible. I felt particularly gleeful seeing him and his new dog because several weeks ago I had put his previous German Shepherd to sleep. She had also been called Martha and was almost identical in appearance to the new version, just many years older. Naming new pets after old pets is a surprisingly common phenomenon. Personally, I cannot imagine ever doing this – to me there was only one Snowy and there will only ever be one Bea. But grief does strange things to people and many clients are only able to cope with the loss of their beloved pet by replacing them with a new identical version. It had been a terribly sad euthanasia as Martha (the first) had end-stage arthritis, and was simply unable to cope any longer despite being completely savvy otherwise. Mr Michael had been brave and stoic but I could tell his heart was broken, so to see him back today under these happy circumstances put a spring in my step. As vets we see the darkest of moments and are there right at the end, but we also see the beginning of life and the development of new and hopefully long-lasting relationships. These are always magical moments.

'She'll be another heartbreaker,' Mr Michael said, giving Martha (the second) an affectionate pat.

'Oh, I know, Mr Michael, but you can't think like that. She's young and healthy and this is the start of a long journey you'll have together. Try not to dwell on the end point.'

'Oh, I didn't mean that. I meant she'll attract all the ladies,' he said, and gave me a cheeky grin.

5 FEBRUARY 2015

A beautiful young tabby cat was brought in by a member of the public today having been found unconscious at the side of the road. We suspected from his injuries that he had been hit by a car, and sadly he died shortly after. I always hate these cases, they make me so sad. Even sadder was the fact that the cat had no microchip and the likelihood was that the owner would never find out what had happened to him. It reminded me of a day back in 2012 when I received a hysterical call from my sister to say that her beloved cat Pixie, whom she had rehomed two years earlier from PWH, had been killed in a car accident. She was contacted at work by a local veterinary surgery who had found her details through the microchip database. Pixie had been brought in by a kind passer-by who had found him on the side of the road, dead.*

I will never forget the anguish in my sister's voice. I drove to meet her and we collected his body and buried him together. It was surreal. He looked perfect, not a scratch on him. He was a stray white and tabby kitten when he first came to us and had lived in our kennels at PWH for several weeks, then with me for a short time before my sister adopted him. I had grown extremely fond of him and he had become my sister's best buddy. We sobbed our eyes out over his grave. However many euthanasias vets perform while wearing our veterinary cloak of self-protection, we are still not prepared for the loss of our own furry friends. When the uniform is off, we are just human beings who love their pets.

I have been asked many times by clients and friends whether they should keep their cats indoors to prevent them from coming to harm. My personal view on this is that cats are free spirits. I have spent many hours of my life watching my own cats chase mice and climb trees and get themselves into bother. Batting at flies in the garden and darting after leaves blowing in the wind. When my friend Mark looked after Bea in his top floor flat for three weeks while I was abroad a couple of years ago, she spent the majority of the time staring longingly out of the window. When she wasn't biting his ankles

*There is currently a petition to make microchipping for cats legally compulsory in the UK as it now is with dogs. In my view the law should also be altered to make it a legal responsibility to report hitting a cat on the road with your car.

at 3 a.m., that is. She was like a caged tiger and would quickly have become deeply unhappy being kept inside indefinitely. So despite the risks, unless a cat has a medical condition, is very elderly or access to the outdoors is not possible, I do think that they deserve the freedom to roam around and explore, and the opportunity to live their best life. I also think microchipping our cats is hugely important. My sister would still not know now what had happened to Pixie if he hadn't been chipped. She would have been left wondering for ever if he was still out there somewhere.

When the member of public, a kind lady in her forties, dropped the cat into the hospital this morning, she commented wistfully as she left that at least he had hopefully had a happy life, even if it was a short one. 'And it's better to burn out than fade away,' she said.

I think she might be right.

6 FEBRUARY 2015

Had a bit of an altercation with a client today about his poor cat Hazel. Mr Welch, a man in his fifties wearing a sleeveless vest on a grey chilly day and smelling strongly of alcohol and cigarettes, arrived late for his morning appointment. He came in with an ice-cold attitude and dragged poor Hazel out of the basket by the scruff of her neck. I immediately disliked him but plastered on my neutral face.

'What's up with little Hazel today?' I asked, giving Hazel a stroke of reassurance.

'She's a total bloody nightmare, that's what's up. Scratches all the time. Leaves hair around the house. Filthy animal. I want rid of her.'

I examined Hazel, a sweet little twelve-year-old tabby cat who had evidence of a flea infestation and large patches of hair loss over her back. Aside from this she appeared healthy.

'Is she well otherwise, Mr Welch?' I asked.

'She's clearly not well; she's shedding everywhere and scratching non-stop. I want her put down.'

'Mr Welch, she's bright as a button and has a treatable skin condition. Have you used any recent flea treatment?'

'I don't want treatment. I've had enough. I want her put down.'

'But she appears healthy apart from her skin disease, don't you think it's worth just trying treatment first?' I pushed. Surely he wouldn't want to put a healthy animal down for no good reason?

'Listen. If you don't do something with her right now, I am going to take her to a field in the middle of nowhere and let her out and then drive off. Or better still I'll find the nearest bridge and throw her in the Thames. I'm telling you right now that's what I'll do.'

Mr Welch was red in the face and sweating by this stage. His voice was raised and his manner aggressive. He hit the wall with his fist and stormed out of the clinic leaving poor Hazel stranded on the table. I popped her back into her box and sat for a minute having a think. We had been reminded by management recently that we were not allowed to admit healthy animals for rehoming. We are an animal hospital, not a rehoming centre, and we don't have the facilities to house endless numbers of strays.

A few minutes later, Mr Welch appeared in the consulting room again having allowed himself some time to cool off. I knew I would get into trouble for this but what choice did I have?

'Mr Welch, I am not willing to put her to sleep, and please don't throw her into the Thames. There are other options available. Would you consider signing her over to us for rehoming?'

'If it means getting rid of her then fine.'

I made a quick call to Esther to explain the situation.

'I'm on my way to you,' she said.

I knew she'd be on my side. Soon enough Mr Welch was provided with forms to sign and an explanation that he would no longer have any ownership rights over his cat, which seemed to please him. How could he own a cat for twelve years and then throw her away like she was an old rag? I could only assume that he was suffering from alcoholism or mental health problems that had made him angry and unable to cope. This thought made his utter distain for his pet easier to stomach. I didn't know his story or what he had been through in his life and I knew I must try not to judge. I couldn't help thinking of all the owners whose pets are gravely ill and suffering but refuse euthanasia and yet here I was persuading an owner of a healthy cat not to put her down. It's a strange job this one, you really never know what will walk through the door next.

At the end of morning clinic I went to visit Hazel settled in her cage in cat kennels. She was a sweet little old lady cat, paddy pawing the bedding as I tickled her chin and raising her bottom and tail in the air as I stroked her back. She would have treatment for her skin issues and then be transferred to one of our rehoming centres as soon as we could find her a space. But from there, who knew how long she would wait in a cage until a kind member of the public came along and offered her a new home. In the world of rehoming animals, this is referred to as a 'forever home', one where she would spend the rest of her days. I could only hope that it would come soon for her and she would feel loved and cherished before long, as every animal deserves to.

9 FEBRUARY 2015

Crazy-but-lovely neighbour messaged this morning to ask if I could help with an injured frog she found in our local park. Luckily by the time I replied poor little Kermit had been gallantly rescued by a passing stranger and placed into the undergrowth in which he hopped away. Thank goodness, as I was about to cancel my day's operations and blue light it straight to the park with my medical kit ready to do mouth-to-slimey mouth if necessary.

10 FEBRUARY 2015

Just seen a client who had purchased an electric shock collar to train his bouncy Jack Russell Terrier, Olive. His neighbours had been complaining about Olive's incessant barking and the owner had tried other methods to train her without success. I'm fairly confident I can speak on behalf of all vets in the UK when I say: please do not use them!

Shock collars in dogs have been used for training or punishment purposes since the 1960s. The idea is that when a dog 'misbehaves', an electric current, activated by a remote control held by the owner, is passed through its collar. The devices are capable of continuously shocking a dog for up to eleven seconds and can send between 100 to 6,000 Volts into a dog's neck. Most dogs will quickly learn not to repeat certain behaviours through fear of further punishment. Sounds more like animal torture to me. Studies have been done by DEFRA to disprove the use of shock collars as an effective method of training and highlight the scarring emotional impact they can have on dogs. Positive reinforcement methods, where dogs are trained by embracing their willingness to please and obey, are always a superior training approach, just as they are with teaching humans. The Kennel Club commissioned a survey in 2014 and the results thankfully showed that the majority (79%) of the public agree that positive reinforcement can improve behavioural issues in dogs and that 74% of the public would like electric shock collars to be banned. I'm fairly appalled that these collars can still be purchased online.* They have already been banned since 2010 in Wales, and Scotland has followed suit. To date, a ban has not yet been put in place in England. Even the thick metal studded collars and chains I regularly see dogs coming in wearing must be terribly uncomfortable. Imagine metal pulling tightly around your throat giving your windpipe a crunching choke every time you get excited or want to play or talk. Of course it isn't always healthy to anthropomorphise our pets, but with regards to training techniques we must try to teach our dogs from an early age how to communicate

*Following widespread campaigning by animal rights activists and animal charities, including the Dogs Trust's #shockinglylegal campaign, the government finally confirmed plans in March 2018 to ban electric shock collars for dogs and cats in England. Boris Johnson even likened the use of the collars to caning a child.

with us, and how to speak our language. If we teach them through aggression rather than patient consistency and encouragement, we can't be surprised when they become aggressive in return. Even a harsh tap on the nose sends the wrong message. Essentially, if you wouldn't want it done to you, don't do it to your pet.

14 FEBRUARY 2015

Just removed a condom from a cat's intestine. The irony of it being Valentine's Day today is not lost on me. I'm just hopeful that the condom had not fulfilled its destiny prior to Sugar the Sphinx chowing down on it . . .

17 FEBRUARY 2015

Winnie came in to see me yesterday as she's not been doing too well. She has had episodes of lameness lately and has been trembling and whingeing at home. She has been very subdued and has not been eating normally. Esther was worried that she was not coping despite the high doses of painkillers she is currently on. I examined her and agreed that she seemed to be very tense. She is a stoical dog and doesn't tend to tell vets when or where she is sore. Never has the phrase 'if only they could talk' been so relevant. If she were a human, I imagine she would tell me that she was in agony today and her right hip was the source of the pain, but that her spine hurt too and she was generally feeling pretty fed up. I could explain in response that bed rest and perhaps even wheelchair use would be our initial plan and that in the long term referral to a psychiatrist and pain management clinic for therapy to help with the emotional scars and chronic pain burden would help. But Winnie is a dog. I was left guessing how she was feeling and hoping that she would respond to twenty-four hours of intense intravenous ketamine and opioid-based painkillers to try and reset her system.

Today I went to visit her in dog kennels where she spent the night on a drip and, despite her clear animosity towards her barking neighbours, she seemed much more comfortable. Thank goodness. She stood up wagging her tail in excitement as Esther approached and we discussed how to proceed. Sarah joined us and three of us stood in front of the kennel trying to make a pain management plan for her that would allow her to continue living the best life she could. The subject of euthanasia lingered distastefully in the air. We all knew it wouldn't be long, although the thought made me queasy. But for now, as long as the good days outweighed the bad, she was off home to be reunited with her furry gang and back where she belonged with Esther.

19 FEBRUARY 2015

As with humans, it's important that animals are healthy and well prior to receiving a vaccination to enable their body to make a good immune response to the vaccine.

Me: So how has Pilchard been getting on?

Ms Smith: Yeah, fine, he's just here for his vaccine.

Me: OK, great, no vomiting, eating well, no general concerns?

Ms Smith: Nope.

Me: [Examines cat, administers vaccination.]

Ms Smith: Although he did have a seizure last week. And he's been drinking more than usual. And he's had diarrhoea for about a month. I think he might have lost some weight. Oh, and he's been pulling his fur out. And last week he vomited but it was just the once. And then again the next day. With blood in it.

Me: [Rocks back and forth in a corner].

23 FEBRUARY 2015

The head of the ambulance department, Amy, brought her cheeky scruffy terrier Ziggy in as an emergency yesterday. They had spent the weekend at the beach and soon after they got home Ziggy had started vomiting and straining to poo. He looked pretty sorry for himself when he arrived at the hospital. I took him straight up for some X-rays and was amazed by the results. Ziggy's entire gut from mouth to bottom was filled with sand. It really was rather an achievement. It transpired that Ziggy loves to dig, and had spent all day on the beach doing so, but unbeknownst to Amy he had also eaten his own body weight in sand in the process. I was immediately concerned because eating that volume of sand can act like cement and cause a serious gut impaction. I performed an enema and, thankfully, twenty-four hours later following some fluids, pain relief and drugs to help the gut keep moving, a repeat X-ray confirmed that the sand was slowly making its way out the other end. He would be pooing out sandcastles for the next three days but he would be OK. Phew.

I have removed a plethora of foreign objects from dogs' and cats' guts over the years, including action figures, plastic bags, corn on the cobs, conkers, a rubber duck, a boomerang, part of a hanger, many plastic teats from babies' bottles, a squeaky pheasant toy, a ball of human dreadlocks, a whole reel of video tape from an old VHS and even a hand-towel from a 60kg Alaskan Malamute called Beast. I often ask myself why they eat these strange things, but no answer is forthcoming. As dangerous as it can be for their health, I suppose these quirks of their character are all just part of their crazy but endearing charm.

25 FEBRUARY 2015

Just seen another client who refused to see me and specifically requested to see my male colleague. I could hear her flirting with him next door with little shrieking giggles. She tried to feed her dog, a Dachshund called Sausage, a cocktail sausage, which slipped out of her hands and fell down her ample cleavage.

'Slippery little sausage, isn't it?' she chortled as she fished it out along with half her breast.

At this stage I got a fit of the giggles, which I had to stifle with a towel that was alas tainted with the smell of anal gland juice from my previous patient. Needs must. One of the nurses saw me and started to laugh too, which simply made things worse and I had to run out of the clinic before the wild snorts were mistaken for a Bulldog on a hot day.

It did lead me to wonder though – why are the male vets I work with so popular? It's true that they are great vets and also lovely caring people, but I don't see what skills they have that make them superior to equivalent female vets. Is it the traditional image of the James Herriot figure?[*] Is it the size and strength that men have on their side? I would understand this more in the farm animal or equine context and I was certainly exposed to my fair share of sexism on farms in my student days being a 5'3" female, but how big do your muscles have to be to lift an 8kg Dachshund?

One of the three members of the senior veterinary team I work beneath at PWH is male. He also happens to be the chief veterinary surgeon. He is one out of only three permanent male members of veterinary staff, compared to the two out of nine female vets currently in senior roles. Thus 33% of the male vets employed are in senior roles compared to only 22% of females. This statistic is actually not too bad compared to the rest of the profession, where there are more than twice as many male vets running their own practice than female equivalents, and more than four times as many male veterinary partners. Sadly, recent surveys have indicated that female vets are more likely to leave the profession or to be disillusioned by their careers, with over a quarter of female vets working part time compared to only 11% of male vets. The Society of Practising Veterinary Surgeons (SPVS) gathers biannual statistics and performs a yearly salary survey on practising vets in the UK. Serial comparisons of male versus female hourly rate have demonstrated a disappointing gender pay gap. The 2014 survey showed a 10% pay gap in favour of men. Female

---

[*]For the young readers out there, James Herriot was a British vet who wrote stories in the 1970's about the animals he treated which were later made into a well-known television series called 'The Yorkshire Vet'.

veterinary nurses were also found to earn less than their male peers.[*]
Inequality is clearly still an issue for many women working within the
veterinary profession. How can this still be the case when the UK vet
schools are churning out female vets in vast numbers? According to
our regulatory body, the Royal College of Veterinary Surgeons (RCVS)
almost 80% of students enrolling in the veterinary degree course are
now female. I would not consider giving my female daughter 10% less
pocket money than my son of the same age. And I certainly wouldn't
be happy if my daughter was less likely to gain opportunities for
career progression or was paid less than a male vet at the same level
and with the same experience as her. Disappointingly, the gender pay
gap in the UK across all professions is above average in comparison to
other EU countries. This in itself may provide some explanation as to
why male vets are so popular in Britain. Members of the public are
used to seeing men in better paid and higher-ranking jobs generally in
society, not just within the veterinary industry. Law, for example, is
attracting an increasing number of women to the profession but
despite this the majority of senior positions at law firms and the judi-
ciary are still overwhelmingly dominated by men.

If male vets are on higher salaries and can more easily progress
further on in their careers than female vets with the same degree of
skills and experience then they must be considered more valuable
to the team. But why? Certainly our traditional shift patterns,
including regular on-call, antisocial and weekend hours and standard twelve-hour day shifts, aren't compatible with family life for
many women, or indeed a good work-life balance for either gender.

---

[*]Fast forward to 2018 and the figures have slightly improved, with no
gender pay gap for veterinary surgeons in the first ten years out of practice. Hurrah! But the pay gap for more senior roles such as partner level
is still significant. Two of the UK's largest veterinary groups were even
identified by the BBC in April 2019 as having the largest gender pay gaps
among UK companies under the headline "Gender pay: fewer than half
of UK firms narrow gap". This is sadly reflective of a profession in
which women struggle to progress as they advance in their careers.

But that does not explain the disparity between hourly rates for male and female vets at the same level. Perhaps it is reflective of women taking time out to have families and then not receiving pay rises or being held back from career progression opportunities when they return. I have certainly heard stories about this happening regularly amongst my female vet friends. I even overheard two male veterinary partners at a conference recently discussing how they do not tend to employ female vets 'of a certain age' because of the possibility they may wish to have a family at some stage soon.*

But in the modern age, many men are also taking career breaks or taking time out to help raise their families, so this must only be part of the story. Perhaps men simply have a greater self-belief and are more likely to ask for pay rises or display their strengths to their bosses, whereas women are more self-critical and don't put themselves forward as often. This is obviously a generalisation and not one that I am able to substantiate with evidence, but whatever the underlying cause, the issue surrounding the gender pay gap in the veterinary profession clearly warrants further investigation.

Women have been a significant part of the veterinary work-force for many decades, with the first female vet, Aileen Cust, becoming a member of the Royal College of Veterinary Surgeons (RCVS) in 1922. Aileen reportedly worked as a qualified vet for 22 years before the RCVS finally acknowledged her veterinary status, going on visits riding side-saddle and volunteering to care for the horses in the First World War. She paved the way for the thousands of female vets that have since followed in her footsteps. Certainly we've come a long way since Aileen's days and I think she would be proud of what female vets have achieved. In 1960 less

---

*A study into gender discrimination within the veterinary profession undertaken in 2018 revealed that, despite taking up 60% of the work-force, female vets still frequently experience gender bias. Interestingly the report, which included 260 UK-based veterinary employers, found that those who believe woman in veterinary medicine do not face discrimination appear to be the biggest perpetrators of equality imbalance and salary disparity.

than five percent of the profession were female. Less than sixty years later we have achieved a significant female majority. Surely it is finally time to shed preconceptions, banish discrimination and allow women's career advancement to progress at the same rate as men's.

27 FEBRUARY 2015

I've performed a grand total of eight ferret spays so far in the last three days. Another animal charity did us a favour a while ago rehoming a bunch of stray terrapins and so when they approached Sophie at New Hope for help with thirteen stray ferrets, she felt obliged to reciprocate. Each day she has been bringing three or four of them to the hospital for neutering, in addition to Diego who is not impressed with his new travelling companions. I dread to imagine the stench they produced on the train at rush hour, or the looks she was given by her fellow commuters. Still, on the plus side there are only five more left to go and I've grown quite fond of the little creatures, despite the fact they are all inbred and try to bite me by bending 180 degrees in every direction.

28 FEBRUARY 2015

Before I started working as a vet, I didn't really understand the concept of compassion fatigue. I always thought it was something that would happen to other vets or doctors, but not to me. I certainly didn't realise that many years of seeing sad and hopeless cases and talking to clients with deeply upsetting personal stories day in day out would ultimately lead to a sense of numbness. The empathy is still there. I still care greatly about all my patients and clients. But my emotions are now buried beneath a layer of detached self-preservation.

Today, a cheeky little eight-month-old Bichon Frise called Archie, whom I had seen a week previously for a pre-neuter health check, was brought in on my emergency shift by its owner, carried in a towel. He had been attacked by a Bull Mastiff ten times his size in the park. I have no doubt that Archie had provoked the Bull

Mastiff, but he ought to have picked on someone his own size.

I was busy examining another animal when Archie arrived so the nurse triaged him and took him straight to our emergency room. She called me to assess him urgently. I could hear the owner sobbing in the waiting room. Never a good sign. I made my apologies to the client I was seeing and rushed out to have a look at him. It only took me a moment to realise he was dead. No heartbeat, eyes fixed, dilated pupils. I removed the towel and, despite all the horrors I have seen thus far in my career, I was not prepared for this one. I knew immediately that this would stay with me. He had been eviscerated. His body had been torn in two with the top half of his torso separated by several centimetres from his lower abdomen and hindlimbs. As I reached in to assess the wounds I found myself cupping his bladder and part of his spleen in my hand, and his bowel spilled out on to the table beneath him. I pressed my imaginary self-protective barrier button and choked back the emotion I could feel welling in my throat as I walked down the corridor to call his owner through. How would I explain this to her? She thought he was still alive.

When I got home tonight, for the first time in a while, I sobbed. Large, salty tears blurring my vision. Great shudders and gasps. I was overwhelmed by a sense of how precarious, unpredictable and cruel life could be. Bea seemed to sense that this was not the right moment to pester me for food and she curled up on my lap and started to purr. She is not a lap cat and I can count on one hand the number of times she has done this. How do animals always know? I curled up on the sofa with her and held her tight. These moments with our pets are so precious and it is easy to take them for granted. Half an hour later after I had composed myself and given Bea some serious chin rubs, she remembered that cuddles are only to be given on her terms and bit my hand. Moment over and back to business as usual. I switched the TV on to some mind-numbing rubbish and attempted unsuccessfully to push the image of Archie and the pain he must have experienced in the moments prior to his death out of my mind.

Just another day in the office.

Part 3

SPRING

3 MARCH 2015

Finally finished a busy 12-hour on-call shift during which I saw
Mr Hart, a young man who walked in for an emergency appointment with his friend's dog, a three-year-old Staffie called Nala.
We established pretty quickly that neither he nor his friend had
any paperwork to prove that they were on means-tested benefits,
and probably weren't eligible for treatment in charity practice. By
law, however, every vet has to provide emergency treatment for an
animal they are presented with, or at least ascertain whether they
are fit to travel elsewhere. It turned out that Nala had accompa-
nied Mr Hart to an all-night rave last night (as you do when you
are looking after your friend's pet), and when his back was turned
she had managed to eat a large bag of 'Jelly Beans'. Nala was
now, in Mr Hart's own words, 'off her tits'. I examined Nala and
sure enough she was completely away with the fairies. Huge
dilated pupils, swaying gait, moments of stupor interspersed with
frantic chasing of her tail. She would not have looked out of place
waving a fluorescent glowstick and dancing to some drum and
bass at Glastonbury.

Staying true to my stance of having zero street cred, I initially
assumed that she had eaten a bag of brightly coloured sugary
sweets – not ideal but unlikely to be life threatening. I soon realised however (with a bit of help from Emma, my designated clinic
nurse that day) that the 'Jelly Beans' he was in fact referring to
were amphetamine drugs. Cue my standard slightly frantic google
search followed by a call to our toxicity helpline to establish how
serious this would be. Every time a poison or toxicity case comes

in that we are not familiar with, vets have access to a helpline called the VPIS (Veterinary Poisons Information Service), manned by experienced staff who have access to data of every similar reported case of toxicity, likely outcome and a recommended path of treatment. Pretty handy when you have clients 'accidentally' feeding non-prescription human drugs to their pets on a regular basis.

By the time I came back to the clinic, Nala had eaten a whole tin of dog food and had stretched herself out in the corner of the room, staring intensely at a picture of a feline 'obesity awareness' poster on the wall in front of her, most likely daydreaming about eating said fat cat.

'OK, so it looks like Nala will hopefully be all right, but I will need to admit her straight away to make her vomit any remaining drugs in her stomach and put her on fluids. It's not ideal that you just fed her a tin of food while I was out of the room, Mr Hart.'

'She's got terrible munchies! The truth is, she may have eaten some hash cakes too.'

Seriously?! I may be a boring non-recreational-drug-taking workaholic, but is it too much to ask for owners (or friends of owners) to stick to one drug overdose in their pets at a time?! I called the helpline again, this time to discuss marijuana. Thankfully, a similar course of treatment was required. Back to Mr Hart.

I injected Nala with a fast-acting drug called apomorphine, which would make her vomit up any drugs left in her stomach, and then continued to question him.

'Can we have the details of the actual owner?,' I asked hopefully. It's very important we get hold of him to discuss Nala's treatment.'

'I don't have a number for John, he's away in Jamaica,' he replied.

Definitely not a charity client. But more importantly, who goes on holiday, leaves their dog with a friend and no telephone number to contact them? I had a sudden brainwave – her microchip number! Thank the Lord for microchips. Emma scanned Nala and sure enough there was a chip. She contacted the microchip company while Mr Hart took a seat and I quickly saw the next two emergencies waiting. Emma returned from her phone call looking disappointed, although not altogether surprised.

'Bad news I'm afraid. The microchip number isn't registered to a man named John. It's registered to a lady called Emily Watson in Liverpool and the telephone number for her is disconnected.'

Agh! I strongly suspected that one of the two emergency patients I had just seen had a corn on the cob stuck in his gut and would require surgery to remove it. There were also two cats with suspected blocked bladders on their way down to the hospital and a series of inpatients that needed assessing. I had to get this sorted and fast. I went back to talk to Mr Hart again.

The more he relaxed in our company and opened up, the clearer it became that Nala could just about have eaten any drug available on the streets of London. Whoever her owner was, and wherever he or she was, Nala was now my responsibility. I packed Mr Hart off home, reassuring him I would call him later and only mildly chastising him for leaving home without his wallet and thus being unable to contribute anything towards the cost of her treatment. I led the now vomiting Nala in her dizzy, trippy state upstairs to kennels to see how a ward full of barking sickly dogs would affect her 'riding the wave'. As I walked out and back down to clinic to assess the next emergency I could hear her howling and wondered to myself what a dog, high on a combination of multiple non-prescription drugs, actually experiences. Was she running through fields of rabbits chasing them with never-ending energy? Was she imagining cuddling up with her long-lost owner somewhere warm and cosy (Jamaica perhaps?), or eating her way through an endless supply of pork chops while playing simultaneously with multiple balls in the park? In the middle of a busy and somewhat calamitous on-call shift, I had to admit – life-endangering aspects aside – I was a tiny bit jealous of her.

5 MARCH 2015

Just discharged Nala. She made a full recovery thank goodness. We finally located the owner and spoke to him on his holidays. He was remarkably nonplussed about the whole situation, even when I emphasised the point that Nala could well have died. It crossed my mind, and not for the first time, that there really should be some sort of basic criteria to allow people to own dogs. Caring an iota about them would be one of the essentials. Mr Hart came to collect Nala this afternoon as her actual owner wouldn't be back for another week and he left us a meaty £10 contribution towards the £250 she had cost the hospital. As a registered charity, we do not expect payment like private practices do, although even then it's impossible to retrieve money from some owners. Animals like Nala slip through the charity net all the time. If they are not fit to travel on arrival, as Nala wasn't, then we simply have to take the hit until they are stabilised and well enough to be discharged or referred, regardless of client eligibility. We would never see another penny towards those costs. But on the bright side she survived and I must remind myself that, after all, is what it's all about.

6 MARCH 2015

Mrs Meldrow and her daughter Ms Turner came back for a check-up with Georgie the diabetic cat this afternoon. Georgie was almost comatosed when I took her out of the basket. A quick blood test confirmed that she was dangerously low in blood sugar. She had been overdosed with insulin. Ms Turner hadn't managed to get to her mother's house for three days to give Georgie's insulin so she gave a double dose this morning instead. Bloody buggery. I injected Georgie with some life-saving glucose to buy us some time and had another long and frank conversation with them about Georgie's treatment. It transpired that Georgie had been struggling with arthritis on her back legs and Mrs Medlrow felt that her quality of life had been poor lately despite starting her on treatment for her diabetes. Mrs Meldrow reluctantly opted to have her put to sleep.

She whispered to Georgie that she would be joining her beloved deceased husband Freddy so not to worry, and that she too would be with them both soon. She clipped off some of Georgie's fur to keep in the locket she wore around her neck with her husband's photo in it. The depth of the bond between people and their pets never ceases to amaze me. Nor does the neglectful nature of people's children. As I administered the fatal injection, Georgie gave Ms Turner one last meaningful swipe and her nail got caught in Ms Turner's hand. I tried to conceal the smirk of satisfaction on my face. Cats always know.

9 MARCH 2015

Crufts is over for another year, thankfully. I watched it last night in horror as German Shepherds shuffled along with their sloped backs and dodgy hips and obese Bulldogs snorted and gasped their way around the ring. Even the Pugs in the 'Best of Breed' category (or 'Best in-bred' category as it has been referred to by the media) looked like little round barrels, despite overwhelming evidence that obesity exacerbates their breathing problems. Researchers from Liverpool University who examined images of 1,120 dogs shown in Crufts between 2001 and 2013 concluded that one in four of them were overweight. This included 80% of the Pugs, 68% of the Basset Hounds and 63% of the Labradors in the study. The Kennel Club have long since implemented breed standards for dogs entering the show and have attempted to make changes to their judging criteria, but these seem to be ignored year after year. It is just so wrong.

When I was a child, I loved watching Crufts and seeing all the different breeds of dogs and their proud owners walk around the ring, apparently enjoying themselves. Short and tall, fluffy and furless, athletic and cuddly. It didn't occur to me that any of the animals could be suffering. In the decades since then, welfare appears to have taken a significant turn for the worse with regard to overbreeding and extreme brachycephalism, or perhaps I have just become more educated through my training about what to look out for. Show dogs are considered to be the ideal example of their breed. By promoting overweight dogs that are struggling to breathe, surely we are simply normalising these issues in the eyes of the public? The BBC stopped airing Crufts soon after the *Pedigree Dogs Exposed* programme was aired in 2008. Aside from the brachycephalics, the programme also found the Basset Hound, Mastiff, German Shepherd, Rhodesian Ridgeback and Cavalier Spaniel to be suffering from genetic diseases following years of inbreeding. The BBC requested that at-risk breeds be omitted from the main competitions in the show, but The Kennel Club were unable to comply, claiming it would be 'inappropriate and counter-productive to exclude any recognised breed'. Soon after this, the RSPCA and Dogs Trust withdrew their support for the event and the show has been televised on Channel 4 ever since. In recent years, several newspapers have picked up on the issues surrounding the show, with Crufts being labelled by *The Independent* as a 'spectacle of cruelty' and likened to the 'plot of a horror film'. The *Guardian* has also published articles in support of change, with a recent headline reading 'Stop buying pedigree dogs. Stop breeding them. Stop these awful practices'. Even the *Daily Mail* has questioned 'are pugs adorable little darlings or inbred freaks?', going on to claim that breeding 10,000 British pugs from a gene pool of only 50 dogs has resulted in tremendous cruelty. There is ongoing campaigning among vets to prevent the use of brachycephalic breeds in advertising and for The Kennel Club to alter their breed standards further, or at least for their current standards to be more strictly adhered to. Minor changes have indeed been implemented, but thus far these have not been good enough to protect the welfare of the animals taking part in the show.*

For the first time since records began fifty years ago, French Bulldogs are now predicted to become the most popular puppy born into the UK. The trusty Labrador is finally being knocked off the top spot. I was unsurprised when I heard this as we are seeing more and more of them at PWH, but disappointed nonetheless considering the difference in the two breeds' health and body conformation. The fact that the number of brachycephalic dogs purchased in recent years has skyrocketed is hardly surprising. In addition to Crufts, which attracts more than 150,000 visitors per year, there is regular misuse of Bulldogs in the media, including frequent advertisements portraying them as the perfect pet. Influential celebrities with millions of young followers on social media have deepened the issue by touting their flat-faced dogs. 'Doug the Pug', a Pug in Tennessee with his own Instagram, Facebook and Twitter account, has a rapidly growing fan base not to mention an online shop selling his Pug brand merchandise. Meanwhile YouTube sensation Zoella, who vlogs about her life with her lovely Pug Nala, has more than eight million followers to date.† I would like to think that the online 'celebrity' brachycephlic dogs have been ethically bred to reduce their likelihood of having the more extreme inherited conditions and that the owners did their homework and consulted their vet before purchasing their dogs, especially for first-time dog owners. But my real concern is for the millions of people who go out and purchase a dog on a whim without obtaining impartial professional advice about which breed might

---

*A new guide called the *Breed Watch Illustrated* was created by The Kennel Club in 2018 to be used to help vets and judges identify physical features that should be flagged up as possible welfare issues prior to entering the show. We must of course welcome these guidelines in the hope that the current situation at Crufts will improve, but as with previous attempts at change, I am sceptical that it will actually be enforced.
†In 2018, Doug the Pug and Zoella now have 3.9 million Instagram followers and 11.4 million YouTube subscribers respectively.

be appropriate for them, because they have seen Bulldogs or Pugs on Crufts or on celebrities' blogs and vlogs and think that they look cute.

I logged on to Facebook on the way to work this morning and saw the usual array of anti-Crufts angry posts and articles I often see in the days and weeks following the show. I know I'm not alone in how I feel about it, but despite the huge body of peer-reviewed scientific literature to back up vets' views, many breeders still disagree with us. I imagine they find our opinions on animal welfare uncomfortable, presumably because admitting that these animals are suffering would affect their lifestyle and income, but also because no one wants to be told, or to believe, that they are causing animals harm. It's a controversial topic, that's for sure. But those of us on the front line dealing with the aftermath of irresponsible breeding are becoming progressively disheartened.*Just like a great ocean liner changing course, Crufts and other bodies must slowly come around to the idea that animals should not be bred to reflect our superficial views of beauty. All animals are beautiful and we must not breed them to live unnatural lives of pain and suffering because we think they look better that way. As another week of airway surgeries, Frenchie C-sections, Dachshund spinal disease and Pug eye ulcers looms ahead, I can't help but wonder – why, when our pets love us regardless of our appearance, can't we do the same for them?

*In 2018, all of the leading dog welfare organisations in the UK finally clubbed together to form the Brachycephalic Working Group (BWG). Their major aim is to improve the health and welfare of flat-faced dogs by working to change their anatomical conformation and reducing the rising demand for these breeds. Since forming, they have met with Disney to discuss managing the increased interest in Pugs following release of the film *Patrick* in June 2018, which featured a Pug as the lead role.

10 MARCH 2015

Crazy-but-lovely neighbour just texted me: *What does one do with a dead duck?*

Is it wrong to pretend I haven't seen the text?

13 MARCH 2015

Mr and Mrs Hasham, a hard-of-hearing couple with their six-year-old Staffie, Boss, came to see me today. Boss has a recurrent seasonal skin condition, which we have been treating for several years, and it has recently flared up again. We managed to communicate through our usual combination of them lip-reading, me doing bad attempts at some sign language, and all of us writing down occasional phrases. At the end of what I perceived to be a relatively successful consultation, I asked them to bring Boss back for a recheck in two weeks' time. I asked this by sticking two fingers up and then quickly realised I was swearing at them. Mr and Mrs Hasham have a wonderful sense of humour and luckily found this hilarious rather than offensive and gently mocked me by both sticking two fingers up at me, and then at each other. At that moment I suddenly realised that we were being watched. I turned around and saw our hospital manager Simon showing one of our big financial donors around on a tour of the hospital just in time to witness the three of us merrily standing swearing at one another. Might be time for me to attend an official sign language course . . .

16 MARCH 2015

Just received a text message from my good friend Kate from university asking me whether I have decided to change my name to 'doctor'. Earlier this month the RCVS made a ruling that vets in the UK will be allowed for the first time to call themselves doctors. Until now, all 20,000 vets in the UK have been 'Mr', 'Mrs', 'Miss' or

'Ms', despite spending five years training at university for a medical degree akin to human medicine in its academic difficulty and postgraduate recognition. 'Doctor' is actually an academic title, which is used as a designation for a person who has obtained a doctorate, i.e. a PhD. Medical practitioners use the term as an honorary title. Traditionally, vets are surgeons, and have therefore been considered 'misters' (and equivalent titles for females) in the UK in the same way that human surgeons revert from 'doctor' to 'mister'. But this concept is out of step with the rest of the world where vets are known as doctors. A change in nomenclature brings us in line with our international colleagues and also allows women to keep their marital status confidential if they wish.

Now that the situation has presented itself to me, however, the decision to change my name seems somehow insincere. All these years after graduating, I have become accustomed to being a 'Miss' or 'Mrs', and being elevated to a new position without any change in academic qualifications seems like I'm pretending to be something I'm not.

Kate wrote in her message, interestingly, that she has noticed how many more of her male veterinary colleagues have already adopted the title relative to her female colleagues. As I contemplated this, I thought again about the fact that men are overrepresented in positions of authority in the veterinary sector. Perhaps male vets feel more confident and comfortable in their roles as veterinary 'doctors' compared to women and so can willingly and more easily adopt the title they deserve.

I asked James his opinion and the answer made me chuckle.

'Of course you should change your name. You've earned it. You should have been a doctor from the start. But of course, technically you're not a real doctor like me.'

James, who is afraid of blood, has a PhD in eighteenth-century German comedy.

18 MARCH 2015

I had a harrowing day today filled with illness and death. By lunchtime, I had already performed three euthanasias, each one sadder than the last. The first two were terminally ill patients whose owners had both lost family members recently and were already in the throes of bereavement. The third animal was owned by a man with a brain tumour who was no longer able to carry his arthritic elderly Labrador up the stairs to his flat. There is something about watching a tough and stoical middle-aged man sitting sobbing on the floor, crushed by the loss of his best friend, that gets me every time. I thought things couldn't get much gloomier but then I checked the afternoon list and realised we had a double euthanasia coming in. It would only be the second one I'd done since I graduated. The first time around both dogs were little old Staffies who had lived together all their lives and had reached a point of deteriorating health simultaneously. The owner and their whole family attended the appointment and it was a sad but peaceful affair. This time around I knew it would feel very different because the dogs I was going to put to sleep were clinically healthy. Sammy and Gunner, one Staffie cross-breed and one Bull Mastiff, had got into a disagreement with the owner's third dog, a Jack Russell Terrier called Bernie, the day before. Unfortunately tempers had become frayed and they had ripped poor Bernie to pieces. He had arrived still alive but there was nothing we could do for him – he was in agony and had severe injuries all over his body, both external and internal. He died shortly after.

Bernie's owner, Mr Floyd, decided today that he wanted his remaining dogs to be euthanised on the grounds that he could no longer trust their behaviour around other dogs or, more worryingly, his grandchildren. Mr Floyd arrived just after lunchtime and the mood was immediately subdued. He was shown to our 'quiet' room with the dogs where they spent twenty minutes sitting on the sofa together saying goodbye before the procedure commenced.

When I came to join them my heart sank. Sammy and Gunner were both young dogs and full of energy and life. They came bouncing up to me, tails wagging, happy and content. I sat down and joined Mr Floyd. I asked him about their general behaviour and whether he had considered behavioural training or rehoming. He replied that the dogs had been rescued from someone who mistreated them as puppies and now lived with him and his two grandchildren. Initially they all got along, but more recently they had been exhibiting aggressive behaviour towards one another and his grandchildren, especially around food or toys. He was struggling to keep them apart or monitor them at all times around the kids. He felt the dogs saw the children as beneath them in the pack and was worried they would be attacked. He also explained that he had called several rehoming centres who had not agreed to take them on because of their history of dog-to-dog aggression. I knew deep down that even if I managed to find them a rescue centre space somewhere, if they failed the behavioural testing (which was likely given the current situation), they would most likely be euthanised anyway. With a heavy heart I printed off consent forms for the owner to sign, discussed the process of putting them to sleep and the cremation options, and then went to fetch the necessary drugs.

The name of the drug used to euthanise dogs and cats is pentobarbitone. It is in a group of drugs called barbiturates, which slow the activity of the brain and nervous system. The drug has been used in humans to treat insomnia, seizures and as an anaesthetic agent. It is also commonly used to euthanise animals in the UK and as a human euthanasia drug in the Netherlands. It is used to execute death-row inmates by lethal injection in several states in America. Interestingly, I am anti capital punishment but it did occur to me that euthanising Sammy and Gunner on the grounds of their bad behaviour was a very similar human-instructed punishment, just in a different species. Did this make it acceptable? I have to hope so, or it makes my job too difficult to bear.

I have become very used to euthanasias. They are part of my everyday working life. But despite this, the process of putting a healthy animal to sleep is always distressing no matter how much I try to rationalise it. I knew that if I refused to put them to sleep, which legally I could quite easily do, I would never forgive myself if a member of the public or one of the children living with the dogs was harmed. Or, even worse, killed. The owner was reaching out to me and asking for my help. The time for educating him about training and behaviour had passed, and there was now only one sensible course of action.[*]

Frieda, my clinic nurse that day, helped me to restrain them and I administered sedation to make them sleepy enough that they weren't aware of what was happening. Mr Floyd cuddled them and told them he was sorry and that he loved them. He then left the room as he was unable to bear the sadness, and I proceeded to inject each dog with an overdose of pentobarbitone until their hearts stopped beating and their chests stopped moving. And just like that, they were gone.

On my way home I used my commute as an opportunity for a spot of self-reflection and to dissect the day's events in my mind. I started to think about my relationship with euthanasia and was cast back to the first one I ever witnessed from a veterinary perspective.

I was a vet student and was shadowing an equine vet. We went out to a call to see a twenty-year-old sweet little chestnut mare called Elsie. She had had ongoing lameness issues in her forelimbs for many months and her owner could no longer ride her as a result. She could not afford to keep her if she couldn't ride her and she felt Elsie was suffering.

---

[*]A study published in the journal *Animal Welfare* in July 2018 based on data from 264,000 dogs in the UK found that one in three dog deaths under the age of three years occurs due to 'undesirable' behaviour such as aggression resulting in euthanasia or poor recall leading to traffic accidents. Clearly, we still have a lot of work to do in the UK to improve dog socialisation and training.

Before I knew it, the vet I was shadowing was reaching for the gun in the back of his car. I had never even seen a gun before and the sight of it made me shiver. I didn't grow up on a farm or a country estate where having a gun licence is commonplace. I grew up in a city, and in the city, guns equal crime and violence. No one I grew up with had a gun or had, to my knowledge, ever seen one either. We had been taught at university about how to use one to euthanise a cow or a horse. How to position it and to pull the trigger by drawing an imaginary X on their forehead and then aiming at the middle of the X so that you didn't end up with a half-dead animal running around a field after you'd fired. But knowing I would probably go into small animal practice, I had never really anticipated being in a situation where I was involved in a death by shooting. Horses are not small animals either. They have bulk. After some sedative drugs were administered by injection, sweet and gentle Elsie was then led into the middle of the field. For one terrifying moment I thought the vet was going to pass me the gun, but in hindsight this would not only have been illegal, but also reprehensible. Thankfully, he told me to stand back and without even so much as a countdown, there was a 'BANG' and she dropped.

It was the convulsions and the volume of blood that came out of the tiny hole in her head that I was not expecting. And standing there in the field, I began my long and gradual process of desensitisation to animal death. I tried hard to act completely normally, because that is what vets do. We put on a brave face and support the owner and swallow our own emotion. But the truth is I was slightly appalled by what I had witnessed, and couldn't help making a species comparison. Imagine shooting a human being under controlled and legal conditions because they were lame on their legs. It suddenly seemed so bizarre. Since Charles Darwin's first descriptions of animals experiencing emotions such as joy, love and pain, anthropomorphism has been regularly demonstrated by humans towards companion animals. But in an age where our domestic pets have now become our family members, is an animal's life still worth less than a human's life? Sadly, the answer does seem to vary depending on the species of animal in question.

All these years later I must have performed hundreds of euthanasias, although thankfully I use a lethal injection instead of a gun. I'm not sure it makes any difference to the animal, but it certainly does to me, not to mention the owner. One Easter Friday on-call ('Black Friday' as I tend to call it), I did twelve euthanasias in one day. I think that's probably my record. They are almost always sad affairs filled with tears and stories of the years of happiness (if the animal is lucky) that have preceded that moment. Many clients comment to me during euthanasias that they wish they could die before their pet so they don't have to say goodbye, or that they would do anything to have just one more day with them. But the truth is that no amount of time with them is ever enough. As a vet, you learn to become detached. It is the only way to cope with the weight of it. Most clients want a strong, compassionate but ultimately unemotional veterinary professional helping them to say goodbye to their beloved pet, and although many times I have shed a tear after doing 'the deed', it is always in private once the client has left.

I checked my phone as I got off the tube and Frieda had texted me to see if I was OK. I feel so lucky to work with the vets and nurses I do, always looking out for one another and providing the emotional support to get through some of the more challenging days. I knew I would walk through the door tonight and be monosyllabic and I would bring down the mood as I explained to James why I was feeling so sombre. This job can be such a rollercoaster and many vets find comfort in forming long-lasting friendships and relationships with one another because of it. The job takes its toll on your private life if you let it. The trick is to try to separate work from life as much as possible, but it's not always easy, and after many years of trying I am still pretty rubbish at it. I think part of the reason I was drawn to James initially was because he represented something completely different to the all-consuming nature of being a vet. He was artistic and creative and non-scientific. He had spent his life learning about art and languages and history and cooking while I had been busily burying my head in veterinary textbooks. He could complete a cryptic crossword in the time it took me to read the first clue, and could answer every question on every programme of *Who Wants to Be a Millionaire?*; it is now one of my life's missions to persuade him to enter this programme and win us a small fortune. But yet he had no clue what any organ in the human (or animal) body was. Years later I still mock him regularly that, despite his many qualifications and intellect, he had no idea what the pancreas was before we met. Living with someone who is remote from the intensity of veterinary medicine makes switching off at the end of the day a tiny bit easier for me because I am unable to obsess about the minutiae of it all. It helps to draw me out of my almost impenetrable fog on days where euthanasias or sad cases weigh heavy on my mind. I am grateful every day that I have James and my family and friends to help me through this crazy whirlwind of vet life. I couldn't do it without them.

19 MARCH 2015

Just seen Katy Purry, a one-year-old female Persian cat and her owners Mr and Mrs Green. Persian cats, along with other flat-faced breeds of cat, have been bred for looks over health in a similar manner to brachycephalic dogs. Unfortunately, this leaves them prone to health issues related to their short nasal passages and compressed skulls, including blocked tear ducts that lead to continually runny eyes, breathing problems that result in snuffling and snorting, and poor dental conformation.

> **Me:** So how's Katy Purry been getting on since I last saw you?
> **Mr Green:** Yeah, great!
> **Mrs Green:** Not good actually, she's back to that sniffling again and the weepy eyes.
> **Me:** OK, let's have a look at her. [Examines cat.] Yes, her eyes are sore again today, aren't they. Any sneezing or coughing?

Mr Green: No.

Mrs Green: Yes, Adam, she has been. [Gives her husband an irritated sideward glance.] She's been sneezing every day and has some green snot coming out of her nose.

Me: And how about her appetite? Does she seem well in herself?

Mr Green: Well, I think she seems fine, she's been chowing down on her Sheba pouches.

Mrs Green: Stop answering for me! You don't actually spend any time with her, do you? She hasn't eaten a thing for two days.

Mr Green: [Mouths 'yes she has' to me behind his wife's back.]

Me: I see. She doesn't appear dehydrated, which is great. Let's just check her temperature. [Places thermometer where the sun doesn't shine.] And she doesn't have a fever either. She does tend to get these recurrent bouts of runny eyes though, doesn't she? And with her breed she finds it difficult to breathe when she gets very snuffly. Is there anything particularly stressful in her environment that could have brought this episode on?

Mr Green: No.

Mrs Green: His family are staying and she hates them. And they hate her too, don't they, Adam? They leave soon, thank goodness. To be honest, I didn't want them to visit in the first place.

Mr Green: [Shoots me a withered look.]

Me: OK. Well for now she can be treated as an outpatient. Keep her warm and offer her plenty of tasty food and fresh water. I'm going to give you some medication for her eyes and we will recheck her in a few days.

Mrs Green: What exactly is the cause of the problem?

Me: Well, because of her breed she has quite runny eyes anyway, and she finds it hard to drain her tears. But I suspect she is also a cat flu carrier, and her symptoms are more extreme because of her prominent eyes and flatter face. Cat flu itself is often viral. Herpes—

Mrs Green: Herpes!! Like the one humans get? That's disgusting!

Me: Or chlamydia. But—

Mrs Green: Chlamydia! And Herpes! Are you saying she's a little tart?

Mr Green: Of course she's not. For goodness' sake, let the doctor speak. And anyway, she's been spayed. She couldn't have sex even if she wanted to, could she, doctor?

Me: Um, these infections, although similar to the human ones, aren't exactly the same. They aren't transmitted by cats having sex. They are usually caught through direct contact with another infected cat that is showing signs of cat flu, which may have happened when she was a little kitten. Then she carries them inside her and that's why she gets recurrent bouts from time to time, usually at times of increased stress. Anyway, she's an indoor cat now, isn't she?

Mr Green: Yes.

Mrs Green: No.

20 MARCH 2015

I went to a pub quiz with some friends tonight. My general knowledge is definitely subpar and I could barely answer a single question. This is a constant disappointment to James. I spend my life hoping random useless facts I have learned at vet school will come up, such as the fact that horses have no gall bladder, rhododendrons make cows projectile vomit, snakes have one lung and two penises and the sneezing distance of a cat is 3.2m (how they calculated this last fact I will never know). Sadly, none of these even came close to being the correct answer to any of tonight's questions about modern culture, politics, sport or history. One day I will win, and then my brain full of useless facts will reign triumphant. Until that day comes, just be aware that Chinchillas have the highest fur density of any land mammal with 20,000 hairs per square centimetre, cats have barbs on their penises, and female camels ovulate every time they have sex. Oh, and pigs ejaculate 250ml each time they get happy compared to only 2ml in humans, just in case you were wondering. I learned that last fact while leaning my whole bodyweight against a sow's back when I was working at a pig farm as a student, trying to 'emulate' the pressure of a boar during intercourse so that she would stand still while she was being artificially inseminated. There are moments in life where you ask yourself 'how the hell did I get here?' That was definitely one of them.

24 MARCH 2015

Totally and utterly broke this month. Paid my RCVS fees today – that dreaded time of the year that every vet gets caught out by at some stage or other. In order to remain a practising vet, every vet in the UK is obliged to pay a renewable licence fee each year to the RCVS, which stands around the £300 mark. Ouch. Some employers cover the cost of this but many – including mine – don't. You are trundling along, trying to claw your way back from the deep dark depression of post-winter blues. You start to see some daylight at the end of the working day and soon you may even see daylight when you wake up. The chill in the air is lifting ever so slightly, and you don't need to wear your attractive thermals under your scrubs anymore. People on the tube aren't looking quite so suicidal on the morning commute (though still a long way from cheery). Life has the potential to be good again. And then bang! You notice that RCVS letter in your pigeon hole and that little bounce in your step suddenly disappears. Why, oh why, I ask myself, do I need to pay to work as a vet every year in addition to all the other expenses, including commuting, extortionate rent in London, compulsory professional development courses and certificate fees? And why does it always come at the same time as my car insurance and car tax and any other large sum of money I am obliged to pay up front? Just to add insult to injury, my toilet also broke this week. Might have to sell a kidney (or a dog's kidney) to pay for that one.

25 MARCH 2015

Just finished a three-hour surgery repairing a cat's intestine after she was shot by an airgun. I could see two pellets on the X-ray but only managed to find one of them during surgery, which had sliced through poor Smudge's bowel and lodged into her abdominal wall, narrowly missing her spleen and left kidney. The second pellet was lodged close to her aorta and could not be located or removed without significant risk of haemorrhage. The aorta is the main artery of the body in mammals and, needless to say, if this vessel is damaged, you're toast. So there it will remain for ever more. Unbelievably, this is the second cat I have seen this month who has been shot. The first cat sadly didn't make it as the pellet hit his lungs. It seems to be happening a lot around London at the moment. I suspect bored and misguided teenagers are responsible. There are currently no laws on airguns in England and Wales and it is no coincidence that this is where 90% of airgun attacks on cats in the UK take place.[*] Laws on airguns are much tighter in Scotland and Northern Ireland.

It does make me wonder what kind of a world we are living in. I hate that people shoot other people and I am definitely a pacifist. But in some ways shooting an innocent cat is even more callous. Animals, like children, have no voice and no strength to stand up for themselves or fight back. They don't deserve to be treated this way. It makes me utterly furious. Go and pick on someone your own size, idiot humans. Or, better still, just go to some anger management classes and take up a hobby that is less likely to maim small creatures. I am going home to console myself with wine and a human voodoo doll. And I'm locking Bea inside

---

[*] A 2016 Cats Protection survey found that 44% of vets had treated a cat which had sustained airgun injuries, and that 46% of those were fatal. Cats Protection has now written to the Home Office as part of their airgun legislation campaign and handed in a petition to Downing Street calling for changes to the laws on airgun ownership in England and Wales.

until further notice, or until her whining by the back door drives me insane, which will probably take about half an hour.

30 MARCH 2015

Just seen six-month-old Hank, otherwise known as a 'bullshit' (a Bulldog crossed with a Shih Tzu). Despite his squashed face, short legs, truncated body and itchy skin, he was kind of cool, and not just because he's called a bullshit. And with a bit of luck, some of his inherited conditions might be watered down by the mixing of gene pools. Either that or he will be double the trouble . . .

1 APRIL 2015

I anaesthetised a chicken today from our local city farm that was possibly egg bound. This means a chicken has an egg stuck somewhere inside her, usually between her womb and cloaca (the communal exit hole in birds for basically everything). It is an emergency condition and can cause birds to die very quickly unless the egg can be removed. Nope, this was not an April Fool's Day joke and was definitely one of the more surreal experiences of my career thus far. I thought it was going pretty well and had just set up the X-ray machine when she suddenly coughed up the tube that had been inserted down her airway to anaesthetise her. With one loud squawk, she bounced up on to her feet in the middle of the anaesthetic, as if nothing had happened.

Having never attempted an anaesthetic on a chicken before, I was a little at a loss what to do after this. I had a good look down below and realised I could see the egg! Her enthusiastic squawk and the anaesthetic drugs must have helped things to move down a bit. It was stuck just beyond her cloaca. The nurse held her wing while I whispered words of encouragement to her and told her to breathe through the pain, which she replied to by pecking me in the face. Fair enough. With a bit of finger assistance and a vat of lubrication, out it popped in all its oval, white, shiny glory. Eureka!

I haven't had that sense of achievement since I removed the grass seed from the Springer Spaniel's vagina a few months ago. Why do all my moments of achievement involve vaginas?

Turns out I needn't have worried about running to Sainsbury's in my break earlier to buy a chocolate Easter egg for James, he could have had the real thing, fried, scrambled or boiled! Though he'd have to get past mother chicken first and I don't fancy his chances. I'm off out for an Easter meal with James's family tomorrow. I might miss out the finger assistance bit when I tell the story.

2 APRIL 2015

I am totally in love with our current rehomer dog Pickle. He is a young male Staffie that was brought in by a member of the public as a stray after a car accident. We have fixed up his broken leg and now he's just sitting here in our kennels as we can't find a space for him in the rehoming centres. Familiar story. Finding kennel spaces for Staffies in rehoming centres is a challenge due to the vast numbers coming through our doors. PWH will never euthanise a healthy Staffie with a good temperament, but equally the centres have to have variety of dogs on offer to attract more potential owners. Staffies sadly often end up staying at the centres longer than other breeds and in my experience they don't tend to cope well in kennels. They can become quickly bored and destructive when left alone for prolonged periods, a phenonenon know as 'kennel crazy', making them even more difficult to rehome. Meanwhile, we continue to be inundated by the breed. Staffies found wandering the streets with no microchip or with a chip that is not registered to an owner. Staffies that have been abandoned in empty properties with no food or water after the owner has moved elsewhere. Staffies who have been tied to lamp posts or left outside the doors of the hospital with handwritten signs around their necks that read, *My name is Rocky, please find me a home*. Staffies with a litter of puppies found sheltering from the rain under a bush. Staffies whose owners have passed away or emigrated or are too poor or too busy to care for them. Staffies, Staffies, Staffies.

Pickle, like many of these dogs, is a handsome cheeky fella with big brown eyes that stare up at you from his kennel in that animal-charity TV advert pulling-at-your-heartstrings sort of way. His tail is a weapon of mass destruction when he's happy, whipping you in the face if you dare to crouch down for a cuddle. He resembles a cross between a Staffie and a dairy cow with big black and white patches, long eyelashes and a dopey grin. Oh, if only I didn't have Bea at home waiting to savage his face upon entry into her territory. I would totally ignore James's protests and bring him home with me! Maybe I will try out taking him home with me next week if he's still with us, that'll be week three in the hospital. But surely he will have a kennel space in a centre and the potential for a forever home by then.

3 APRIL 2015

Sophie came to find me when I was operating earlier.

'Is there a morning-after-pill for pigs?' she asked. I can always rely on her to be completely random.

'Um, I'm pretty sure there are hormonal implants or injections that can be administered to induce miscarriage,' I answered. My porcine reproductive knowledge is not what I would consider 'up to date', having read very little about it since I was a student.

'Why are you asking?' I was slightly afraid of the answer.

'Oh, it's my new pig, Einswein, he's a disaster. He is so randy he's humping everything! Any animal, any species, and he's getting really aggressive with it. One of the volunteers at New Hope just called to say he had locked on to the female pig he was rehomed with and now she has a ton of liquid pouring out of her. The last thing we need is another ten piglets to care for. And we don't even know if they are related; can you imagine if they were born with disabilities and I had to commute on the tube with them each morning *and* Diego . . .'

The thought of ten little piglets on leads sitting next to her on the tube at rush hour made me snort into my operating mask.

'I'll do some research for you. Don't worry, we will get it sorted. But for goodness' sake get Einswein castrated!'

5 APRIL 2015

Easter Sunday on-call:

Vomit-inducing drugs at the ready – check.
Chocolate toxicity calculator app downloaded – check.
Theatre packs sterilised ready for chicken and lamb bone lodged
 in gut removal – check.
Intravenous fluid packs ready to flush out those hot cross bun
 raisin toxins – check.
An abundance of cheap chocolate stashed safely around the
 hospital for staff to munch on – check.

Let's get this party started.

8 APRIL 2015

Came in today to find that Pickle the stray Staffie was up in the isolation ward over Easter to give him a break from all the noise in dog kennels and he had managed somehow, in his distress at being stuck in a kennel alone, to get his penis caught on the kennel door and rip the fleshy part of it right off. Absolutely gutted. I operated and think I did a reasonable job of repairing it but I have never seen anything like it. Penises bleed a lot, as it turns out. Luckily in dogs they have bones down the centre to provide some structure during the surgical repair. My pal Kate turned to me in an anatomy lecture on the canine male reproductive tract in our first year at vet school and asked me whether human males have bones in their penises too. I still mock her about it twelve years later. Sadly, despite said bone, it was still a mushy, bloody mess. I simply can't imagine the agony of it, or the frustration he must have felt to get himself into that situation in the first place. This will delay his chance of getting a kennel space in a rehoming centre even further. I sat with him and got some essential cuddles and face licks before I left work and told him it was all going to be OK. The thing is, I'm not a hundred per cent sure I believe that's true.

9 APRIL 2015

Another penis surgery on Pickle today. I'm becoming quite the expert. All his sutures from the last surgery broke down and the wound became a complete mess. It was almost impossible to cobble it back together again. What he really needs is a specialist surgeon performing some kind of salvage procedure, but instead he has zero budget and zero potential for a new home now. Chances are looking slimmer by the day.

10 APRIL 2015

After a group vet meeting about Pickle this morning we decided reluctantly to put him to sleep. We have been left with no choice. I know we tried our best and probably did more than most other charities would or could do, which is part of the reason I am so drawn to PWH and so passionate about the work we do. But I can't help feeling that he is just another Staffie let down by society and let down by us. Goodbye, my furry friend. Hope you find lots of squirrels to chase up there.

12 APRIL 2015

Glanced down at my phone during lunch with the in-laws today to see a picture message sent to me by Sarah. I knew she was on-call and wondered what it could be. I opened the message to find a picture of a 200kg boar lying upside down on our operating table being castrated by Sarah, with Sophie in the foreground doing a 'thumbs up'. I started to giggle uncontrollably. The kind of laughter that you can't suppress and the more you try, the worse it gets.

'What on earth is so funny?' James asked.

'Oh, nothing.' I quickly shut my phone and did my best to compose myself. Not ideal lunchtime material for the non-surgeons around me currently eating their roast pork.

14 APRIL 2015

I'm having an extremely rare day of feeling entirely competent in my profession and like I can conquer the world after performing my first solo cruciate surgery! Woohoo! The cruciate ligament is an important part of a dog's knee, but relatively commonly it can rupture causing a painful and immobilising injury. It usually requires orthopaedic surgery to repair it, followed by a lengthy period of rest while it heals. I've been training for several months to do the surgery and was extremely nervous as I scrubbed up this morning, knowing that for the first time today I would be operating on a dog's knee alone with no other surgeons by my side for moral support. But now, several hours and one successful surgery later, I'm riding the wave of the surgical high! I'm sure it will be business as usual tomorrow and back to stumbling my way blindly down a path of insanity, attempting to put out multiple fires with a tiny ineffectual drop of water, but for now I will enjoy my brief and self-promoted supervet hero status. I can do it! Grace the Staffie will run across fields chasing squirrels again (possibly slightly stiffer and slower than once she did) thanks to me!

15 APRIL 2015

My bubble has burst. Grace's owner left a £3 donation today when they collected her, towards a surgery that I had spent countless hours after work practising and would have cost a minimum of £1–1,500 in private practice. Our clients are given a breakdown when they leave the hospital containing an estimate of what their pet's treatment has cost us. It is not a 'bill' as such, but they are asked to leave a contribution towards the total amount or cover it in full if they are able to. One hundred per cent of their contribution goes towards the running of the charity – vets individual salaries are set in stone every year in the charity sector and we don't receive bonuses, nor is the job incentivised based on revenue as is the case in many private practices. Sadly, a trend has developed of very small financial contributions being made towards services that would cost potentially thousands of pounds elsewhere and are uniquely offered by our non-government-funded charity. Even in human medicine, orthopaedic surgeries usually cost several thousand pounds, with the NHS forking out £2,900 per person for a broken arm, £5,120 for a broken leg and £5,620 for a hip replacement according to estimates from the Nuffield Trust. Perhaps, however, our amazing NHS is part of the problem in the UK with respect to veterinary fees. Many members of the public are simply unaware of the realistic cost of hospital procedures and surgeries, both for humans and animals. Of course, if clients genuinely have no money then that is what we are here for. But I have become cynical that this is not always the case. And without our service, Grace would most likely have continued to limp on in significant pain for the remainder of her life.

When the unimpressed reception staff informed me about the measly contribution, I tried not to focus on the fact that the client had had two mobile phones, one of which was an iPhone, and had to leave the consultation halfway through as his parking permit had run out on his sports car that was parked outside the hospital. How he was eligible for government financial aid and thus for PWH treatment I don't know, but this is not an unfamiliar scenario. Three pounds! Yesterday's elation was rapidly replaced by frustration and has now, several hours and a glass of wine post-shift later, turned to resigned acceptance. I try so hard to be non-judgemental in this profession, but why is it always the genuinely poorest clients who leave the largest contribution towards the cost of their pet's treatment? It's one of life's frustrating conundrums.

17 APRIL 2015

Asked a client to clarify a dog's age during a consultation today as we hadn't entered it into the computer system properly.

'Oh, he's somewhere between one and twelve.' So, the entire lifespan of the animal then.

20 APRIL 2015

Just seen one of my favourite clients, Ms Cruz and her dog Precious, a little biting cross-breed, half Chihuahua and half Shih Tzu. Ms Cruz had fallen on hard times when she lost her job as a cleaner after her boss cottoned on to the fact that she was refusing to clean cobwebs from the ceilings and windows because she didn't want to destroy the spiders' homes. What a legend.

Four weeks ago, I broke the news to Ms Cruz that Precious had a nasty form of breast cancer. It had already spread to multiple lymph nodes and during today's examination I suspected it had also spread to her lungs. Amazingly, unlike many dogs with cancer I see, Precious had actually gained weight since I last saw her and was looking rather portly. When I questioned Ms Cruz about her dog's appetite she explained that she has been stuffing Precious with every type of food you can imagine in addition to her usual dog food. She listed about ten different types of meat including Precious's new favourite – M&S honey roasted ham with pomegranate molasses. I asked why she had been feeding her so much and her answer was simple: if she feeds Precious more food then the cancer will eat the food and not her dog. The answer hurt my heart. Ms Cruz showed me her notebook in which she had written a chart every day to ensure Precious received all of her medication at the correct times, even if it meant giving her tablets at 3 a.m. On one side was a small column with a drug name I didn't recognise.

'Oh, ignore that one, that's my depression medication,' she muttered.

My heart took another hit.

She lifted her other dog, Eduardo, a six-year-old Chihuahua, on to the table next for a weight check. He has been on a diet for six months for his obesity and thus far has managed to lose a fabulous 50g (equivalent to the weight of one of his poos). As it turns out, Eduardo has been sharing all of Precious's treats, including the delicious and highly calorific honey roasted ham. I took the executive decision on this occasion to ignore the fact that he had gained 300g since the last appointment and reassured her that she was doing a great job. She came around the table and gave me an emotional and slightly winding hug. I don't often have physical contact with clients – even during euthanasias it's usually just an arm pat or brief shoulder rub. But Ms Cruz was different. She thanked me multiple times and then wandered down to our pharmacy to collect more pills for Precious.

In the next life, please can I come back as one of Ms Cruz's dogs? Or, better still, one of her spiders?

22 APRIL 2015

I'm having a 'I need a glass of wine urgently' sort of evening. Thank God Sarah was on standby to accommodate this and we went straight to the pub at the end of our shift. For the very first time in my life I was called a 'bitch' at work today. Perhaps this makes me a lucky individual that the people I have come across so far in my working life have been generally respectful and civilised. Or perhaps I just haven't wound anyone up enough to justify such name calling. Until now.

Ebony is a three-year-old black Staffie that came into the hospital yesterday with a fractured femur (thigh bone). The owner, Miss Belmonte, told me that Ebony had been limping for a month following a car accident. Not just a minor limp but completely lame on her left hind leg and dragging it behind her. A *month*! It still shocks me how long some people will leave their animals before seeking veterinary attention. I'm pretty sure Miss Belmonte wouldn't have left her own leg for a month with a fractured femur before popping down to her GP. Ebony was extremely tolerant of being examined under the circumstances and it didn't take me long to establish that she had a fracture. This was confirmed on X-ray and, after lengthy discussion with my more surgical and orthopaedically minded colleagues, we made the decision that amputation was the only viable option. The fracture had been left for so long that it had started to heal at a bizarre, unnatural angle and we would have to rebreak it to try and mend it. But more concerning than this was the loss of nerve function in the limb, which was highly unlikely to ever return to normal.

I called Miss Belmonte and set about trying to explain the situation. I introduced the idea of amputation gently – it is difficult for some owners understandably to come to terms with their pet needing to have a limb amputated. I would find this very hard if it was my own pet, despite seeing it every day in my job. The owner remained relatively silent and monosyllabic throughout this discussion. I asked if she had any questions, to which the answer was a firm 'no'. I then asked why she had not been able to bring Ebony in sooner. It is part of my job description to protect the welfare of the animals under my care, and had I turned a blind eye to this I would not be fulfilling the oath I took at graduation. All vets in the UK say an oath when they graduate that includes the following: 'I promise . . . that I will pursue the work of my profession with uprightness of conduct and that my constant endeavour will be to ensure the welfare of animals committed to my care.' We are trained to act as an impartial source of information on animal health and welfare issues, and we try our best to do so. I explained to Miss Belmonte that I thought Ebony had been suffering and should have been brought in immediately following the car accident for pain relief and veterinary assessment. The sad truth was that if Ebony had come a month earlier, we probably could have saved her leg.

I could feel the tension mounting on the other end of the phone and knew I was about to receive some unwelcome but predictable client aggression. The combination of a client with a fiery temper, the news about amputation and the guilt of not having brought Ebony in sooner were the perfect ingredients for an explosion. Silence for a second, and then it came. I am used to client rage. I have become hardened to it. I am used to anger and frustration turning into blame, and I am used to being a punching bag. I was expecting it when she said she would refuse the limb amputation, that she didn't trust a word I was saying, that I was meant to care about animals, that I had no idea how busy she had been over the last month and Ebony had seemed fine to her. I was expecting it when she told me she would be going for a second opinion, and then changing her mind when we discussed private practice costs. What came as a bit of a shock, however, was the personal attack that followed.

'You're just a little bitch, that's what you are.'

Wow. Pretty harsh.

'I don't think that language is appropriate,' I limped on with an attempt to pacify her, 'and I will terminate the conversation if you continue speaking to me that way. I appreciate you are frustrated, and I am so sorry that Ebony's fracture is not repairable, but we need to deal with the situation we are now in. We can't leave her as she is.'

'The only conclusion here is that you are a total and utter BITCH.'

She spat the word at me. It was full of malice.

'I'm sorry, but you are. Calling me and speaking to me like this,' she went on. 'You must be a total bitch otherwise you wouldn't have said those things. Looking down your nose at me when really you don't give a SHIT. You claim to care, but you don't. I won't deal with you anymore, I want to speak to someone else who actually cares about animals.'

I ended the conversation by agreeing readily to pass the case to a colleague, though I pitied my poor colleague. I was certain I had behaved professionally and that I had said nothing indefensible. Even my questioning on Ebony's welfare had been relatively gentle. But for the rest of the day I couldn't stop hearing her vicious words in my head. I have been told many a time by owners that I don't care about animals, or that I don't know what I am talking about, as have all my colleagues. These seem to be the default comments when owners don't like or don't want to accept what we are saying. And with the ease and immediacy of social media, many vets are now also plagued by constant online criticism to add to the face-to-face and over-the-phone attacks. Once upon a time I would have defended myself and tried to reason with Miss Belmonte, explaining to her that I do of course care about animals. Her comments would have bothered me and stayed with me at night as I tried to get to sleep. But after a number of years in practice I have become rather numb to the negativity as long as it's not a personal attack on my character. I feel secure in the knowledge that I always do my utmost to protect and care for the animals I treat, and I now have a much greater understanding of people's behaviour and the human desire to lay blame through guilt than once I did.

This time felt different, though. To call me names directly in that manner somehow felt like a violation. It stung. For the remainder of the day I was unable to shed my heightened sense of anxiety and found it almost impossible to unwind. I think many clients underestimate the effect they have on us vets. There is a human behind the uniform after all. We are not impervious, and most of the time we are just trying our best to do the right thing, and to protect and defend our patients who are unable to do so for themselves. Tomorrow is another day and life moves on, but these moments stick with you. You don't forget them.

24 APRIL 2015

We have had not one, but two, stray bearded dragons brought into the hospital this week. One was found on Tooting Common and the other on Hampstead Heath on different days and opposite ends of London. So random. They're pretty cute, actually. We've named them Toots and Heath. My nephew, who has a penchant for anything with scales, was beyond excited when I told him about them and asked if they could come and live with him and their fat cat Gizmo, lizard Spike and hamster Sandy. Considering they are antisocial creatures that do not like being kept together, and each one will require a minimum of a four-foot cage, I think my sister might be less than impressed by this idea.

When I heard that they had arrived, I must admit I was fairly unsurprised. We often have weird and wonderful creatures brought in to us, which is odd considering we are located in the centre of a large city. In 2011 we made the news after admitting a ring-tailed lemur (native to Madagascar, I should add) to the hospital that was found in sub-thermal temperatures on Tooting Common. We named him King Julien after the character in the animated film *Madagascar*. How on earth King Julien made his way to London town from his home 5,700 miles away we will never know, but Tooting is clearly the place to be for exotic creatures. There was some speculation at the time that he was being kept illegally as a pet and had either escaped or been abandoned by his owner.

Unfortunately, findings from freedom of information requests sent to every UK council have found that lemurs are one of the most popular exotic animals being kept as pets, with a suspected 115 lemurs in UK households. Sadly, this information also revealed that pumas, alligators, crocodiles, poisonous snakes and even tigers are being held captive in homes throughout Britain. Wild animal licences are meant to only be granted to people who have the required safety measures in place and keep these animals for conservation or breeding purposes, such as zoos or wildlife sanctuaries. Clearly, this is not always the case.

After some frantic googling we established what food he might like to eat and set about making him feel comfortable in his new home in our (luckily empty) isolation ward while we tried to work out what on earth to do with him. I was the unlucky vet on-call that weekend and always cringe when I remember the moment the film crew showed up to ask me questions for the news programme he was being featured on. I was in-between emergency surgeries at the time, so I raced down to clinic, mumbled something about how lemurs are not native to the UK, and that King Julien had luckily warmed up and managed to eat some honey from a syringe, and then I raced off again. It was only as I ran up the stairs that I caught a glimpse of myself in a mirror and realised I had been interviewed for national television wearing my surgical hat with hair poking out in a ninety-degree angle and a deep crease across my nose from my surgical mask. Oh well, no time for vanity in this job.

King Julien luckily survived and was transferred to a wildlife centre to find a home. I'm hoping Toots and Heath will also do well and be taken on by someone who knows how to care for reptiles. It does worry me, though, that these intriguing exotic creatures frequently end up in the hands of people who have no idea how to look after them. They need special care, which is often neglected when the novelty has worn off, not to mention the potential threat to the public when the more dangerous species escape. From here on I'm certainly going to watch my back when walking across Tooting Common at night.

26 APRIL 2015

It's the London marathon today, and I'm on-call. Really hope the distraction of the runners keeps things quiet. My sister called me last night and we were chatting until late so I'm feeling pretty tired. She asked my advice about getting a dog and which breed I would recommend. It's always a tricky one when people ask me this. As it was a family member, I let my thoughts spill out in a haphazard fashion without holding back. I realised after about forty-five minutes that I had barely paused for breath. I guess working in this job gives you a skewed view of the different health ailments each breed gets. A huge part of our job is pattern recognition and knowing what likely diseases might affect certain animals, so much so that my friend and line manager at work, Jane, wrote an entire book about breed predispositions to disease in dogs. I see so much illness and, when I think about it, not very much health. Some breeds that are particularly prone to health conditions even have diseases named after them, such as 'Shar-pei fever', 'Westie lung' and 'Boxer cardiomyopathy'. The nurses do a lot of the routine vaccinations and, in an average week, of the 50 to 100 animals I see, only a handful of them are actually healthy. So when my sister asked me this, despite loving dogs of every shape and size, I struggled to think of any specific breed of dog that I would recommend without worrying about the problems that they could develop.

'What about a Labrador?' she asked.

'Well, they're certainly good family pets so would be great around children if properly trained. You'd have to put an awful lot of energy and time into training and socialising early on – though that goes for any dog – but also I would definitely get one from a breeder that has them hip scored. They can be so debilitated by hereditary hip and elbow dysplasia.' I went on to explain to her that hip and elbow dysplasia are inherited conditions caused by abnormal formation of the joints, leading to lameness and painful arthritis. They are sadly very common in large breed dogs with as many as 18-49% of German Shepherds and 17-21% of Labradors being affected, compared to 0.72% of dogs overall.

'Right. What about a flat-coated or Golden Retriever? They're beautiful dogs.'

'They are prone to cancer of the lymph nodes and spleen. And have the same issues with hips and training requirements as Labradors.'

'Oh, OK.' She sounded a little deflated. 'A Staffie?'

'They're great with kids when well trained,' I replied, trying to sound upbeat. 'Although they are very prone to hereditary skin disease and not always great with other dogs. And they are full of beans so you have to put in the hours walking and training them.'

'Ooh, a German Shepherd? I've always wanted one of those!'

'Definitely not as your first dog. They can be absolutely fabulous pets, but you need to know what you're doing. They can be quite nervous if not handled and trained correctly. And they get bad hips. And horribly infected skin around their anus,' I added for good measure. *

'Ew, gross. OK. Well, what about a smaller one. A Spaniel or Terrier?'

'Cocker Spaniels are lovely but nutty and high maintenance and get yeasty ears and feet. Cavalier King Charles Spaniels are super cute, I rarely come across one that has a bad attitude. Great with kids.'

'Oh, OK, super!'

'But they tend to die of heart failure and have squished brains,' I added.

'Maybe not then.'

'Terriers can be great pets!' I piped up again. 'They are quite headstrong, and you have to be careful with them around children as they're not always hugely tolerant.'

'My friend had a miniature Dachshund, it's so cute! What about that?'

'Sure if you have a spare five thousand pounds to spend on spinal surgery when the time comes.'

'Pug?'

'Don't even get me started. You'll love it with every fibre of your being but will be bankrupt and heartbroken within six months.'

'Well, tell me what breed you think we should get then!' she

---

*German Shepherds are unfortunately prone to a condition called anal furunculosis, a chronic inflammatory disease resulting in ulceration and inflammation surrounding the anus. It's essentially a big, red, painful arsehole.

said, slightly exasperated. I realised I hadn't thus far been particularly helpful.

'Would you consider a Heinz 57 from a rescue shelter?' I asked.

She said that yes, she had considered this, but was worried that a dog she hadn't known from puppy-hood may not be a hundred per cent trustworthy around her young son.

'Yes, I can see that's a concern. But many of the dogs in rehoming centres have grown up with kids and are put through behavioural assessments to make sure they are matched up with suitable homes. You could go and visit one of the centres and meet some of the dogs and see what you think?' I offered.

'OK, well, it's something to think about. If I did decide to get a pedigree, though, do you think it'd be OK to buy a puppy from an online breeder?'

'No! Definitely not! So many backyard breeders using and abusing their dogs like commodities advertise online. You'll end up with a really sick little puppy. No, no, no! You must make sure you see the breeding environment and ideally both parent dogs, or at the very least the mother dog in person.'

I'm pretty sure my sister was a bit fed up after this as she changed the subject soon after. In hindsight, perhaps I was a bit doom and gloom. It's so difficult to step out of the vet shoes when you're asked your opinion about purchasing a new pet by friends or family members. I absolutely love dogs but I can't bear them suffering unnecessarily. As a charity vet, it's not that I am anti-pedigree, or anti-breeding. Some of my favourite patients are snuffly Pugs and Staffies with terrible skin, despite their health ailments. Someone somewhere has to breed dogs or they will become extinct. But I have just seen so much terrible and irresponsible breeding.

Canine domestication began around 15,000 years ago so we have been influencing their breeding for a long time. Their bond with humans is absolutely unique; even horses haven't learned to understand and communicate with us in quite the same way. Dogs are special creatures and we are privileged to be able to live alongside them. But since we have been breeding show dogs, I just don't feel confident recommending many of the pedigree dogs out there to an average family, especially one with no previous experience with dogs and a limited budget to spend on their care.

I suppose when advising my sister I was trying to protect her from any future financial and emotional upheaval. Although on the bright side she could end up with a German Shepherd that doesn't have hip dysplasia, or a Cavalier King Charles Spaniel (Cavie) with a healthy heart, especially if she finds a bona fide breeder. I guess you have to take some gambles in life. I would struggle to choose one pedigree as my own personal favourite, although scruffy terrier breeds such Border Terriers would be high on my list. I love their cheeky little characters and their curly, coarse coats. Border Terriers are generally a popular breed among vets, partly because they are small enough to come to work with us or be ferried around in a car when doing farm animal or equine calls. I do also go gooey for a soppy 'please tickle my tummy immediately' Labrador, although I think Cavies top the charts for the kindest and most patient temperament. They are incredibly gentle souls, despite their often broken hearts. And then there are Staffies. Bouncy, jubilant, attention-seeking, energetic and endlessly enthusiastic Staffies. Wherever my future career takes me, they will always now have a place in my heart. That enormous grin with their tongue lolling out to one side and their absolute frenzied need to love and be loved. They are, quite simply, wonderful. But pedigrees aside, my overall favourite type of dog is, and always will be, a good, old-fashioned mongrel. You just can't beat them.

I checked the day-list before lunch to see how the afternoon was looking. First three appointments:

Benny, seven-year-old Cavie – recheck heart problems.
Sarah Jessica Barker, two-year-old Staffie – skin red raw.
Oliver, three-year-old Dachshund – off his back legs.

#adoptdontshop[*]

28 APRIL 2015

Saw a Staffie back for his recheck appointment today who I had seen the day before with vomiting and diarrhoea. I had made the standard recommendation of feeding small bland meals of chicken and rice.

Me: Did you try the chicken and rice?
Owner: Yes, but it hasn't worked, he still has the squits.
Me: What exactly did you feed him?
Owner: We shared a bucket of chicken from KFC.
Me: [Bangs head repeatedly against a wall.]

1 MAY 2015

Been rooting for a little baby crow this week who was found struggling to walk on a sore foot and brought in to see me on my on-call shift. He has been affectionately called Crowella Deville by the receptionist who registered him. We have so many birds brought in by well-meaning members of the public, but sadly they would often be much better off left to their own devices, especially the baby birds. They can look unsure of their footing and can be easily caught when they first explore outside of their nest by people who think they are poorly and in need of veterinary assistance. And once they have been brought to us we are never able to

---

[*]Since writing this diary entry my sister has indeed adopted a dog. A wild and wilfull (though also gorgeous and loving) partially-sighted German Shepherd cross Collie, aptly named Luna the lunatic. So glad she took on board all of my advice . . . To be fair she adopted the crazy loon through Sophie's charity so it's Sophie I blame each time I receive a new text from my sister about how Luna's eaten another hairbrush or won't stop barking at the neighbours . . .

reunite them with the mother bird, who must be beside herself looking for her young. It has given me a new appreciation for the term 'empty nest syndrome'. The baby birds we see often call and pine for their mum for days or even weeks after they arrive, if they survive. And many of them perish without their mother to care for them, despite our best efforts.

Of course, most of the birds brought in to us are an array of London's finest pigeons. Pigeons with clubbed feet, damaged beaks, torn feathers, twisted wings, covered in flat flies and scabs and with a feisty desire to live.* They are tough little things and, if you look past their ubiquity, they are also rather beautiful. We have a limited budget to help wildlife but we always do what we can, within reason. One client who carried a sick pigeon in to us in her Prada handbag proceeded to call us eight times during emergency hours to enquire about said pigeon. Unfortunately, I had had to euthanise it soon after it arrived at the hospital (around the time of phone call number five). She then put in a complaint to head office because I had not been able to save it. She was displeased that we hadn't tried harder, used more of our time and resources to help it. Of course I had tried, but sadly we can't save them all, and when they have broken wings or deep bone infections they simply won't survive back out in the wild.

Crowella Deville is a little bit special though. Almost as special as Steven Seagull, a handsome seagull I became similarly fond of last year, who had lost his way from his chip-stealing antics on Brighton pier and found himself stranded among crowds of people on Oxford Street. Unlike the mighty Steven, though, Crowella is quite tiny still

---

*Flat flies are pigeon louse flies that have adapted to clinging to and moving through pigeons' plumage by developing a flat body and specialised claws. They feed on pigeons' blood and are particularly unpleasant little things. I have seen a group of unshockable veterinary nurses running around hysterically screaming in disgust as a flat fly flew off a pigeon and chased them around the room.

and sits on my shoulder in a Johnny Depp Captain Sparrow pirate fashion while I assess his chart and he squawks at me for food. His foot is still infected but he's off to a wildlife centre we are affiliated with later today who have the facilities to nurse him back to health before he is set free again. He is a cutie and I am not normally a bird fan, based largely on their fragility and potential to drop dead from shock at any given moment, combined with my own lack of avian knowledge. I hope he makes it and is flying around the Tower of London again before long with his other crow pals.

2 MAY 2015

I performed one of my favourite surgeries today – a C-section on a stray Staffie that was brought in yesterday by a member of the public. She had very saggy teats and looked around four or five years old. I suspected she'd been used as a breeding bitch, churning out puppies for a backyard breeder or on a puppy farm. She'd had a lucky escape. Unfortunately, she went into labour early this morning but got into trouble and needed urgent surgery. I tend to prefer medicine to surgery as I find the drama and unpredictability of operating unsettling. But despite being a complex and tricky surgery, there is nothing quite like the sight of little tiny puppies wriggling around inside a womb as you cut them out and free them into the world.

I also love the camaraderie of it. With a nurse on anaesthesia and two on standby to receive the puppies, it always feels like a real team effort. The nurses vigorously rubbed each of the tiny wriggling balls of newness in towels and ensured they were breathing and warm while I continued to operate on the mother dog. I spayed her at the same time prior to her transfer with her little ones to a rehoming centre. Her days of being used and abused as a puppy machine were over.

I went to visit them at the end of my shift all snuggled up together in their kennel. News of the new Princess who Kate and Wills have named Charlotte (good choice) has just hit the headlines. Seems they stole my dog's thunder. I checked the puppies' genders – three boys and two girls. I smiled as I wrote their new names on the file: William, Harry, George, Kate and Charlotte. And as for the mother dog – Queen Elizabeth. Obviously.

4 MAY 2015

Just seen two twelve-day-old puppies, one of which was semi-comatosed. The owner walked in with her children, a little boy of around six and a girl of around four years old. I asked her what had happened and she explained that her son and his friend had been 'playing' with the puppies downstairs while she was upstairs with her daughter. Apparently the friend had suggested they try throwing the puppies against the wall for fun. The son had been reluctant, but the friend picked up the male puppy and threw him. He copied with the little female puppy but apparently with less gusto. By the time the owner came down to find them, the female puppy was stumbling around in a daze and the male one was collapsed and unresponsive.

I admitted the puppies for treatment immediately, trying to suppress my deep rage. I have seen very sick puppies and kittens rally before following head trauma. Our head nurse ended up adopting a cheeky little ginger kitten called Woody that had arrived unable to walk after he had been shut in a door. I thought he would survive less than twenty-four hours but he's still going strong seven years later. However, the truth is it's not always a happy story, and depending on the degree of trauma, there could be permanent brain damage at best, or a progressive coma leading to death.

An X-ray revealed a skull fracture on the little male puppy. The force it must have required to cause this degree of trauma was shocking and I struggled to get the image of the little boy throwing the tiny little helpless puppy weighing only a couple of hundred grams out of my mind.

Using a great deal of willpower, I purposefully stuffed my rage back into the emotional black hole where most of my feelings of frustration and exasperation go during the course of a working day. Rage wouldn't help this puppy, or help to educate his owner. Nor was I able to educate the other child belonging to someone who wasn't even one of our clients. But I knew that ultimately the issue lay with the owner who left the boys unattended with the puppies in the first place. I went back to talk to her and she seemed thankfully very remorseful. The little boy hid his head in her coat as I spoke and had clearly been chastised for his crime. I tried to speak slowly and calmly as I explained to the mother and her children about their duty of care to their pets, and that puppies are fragile just like new-born babies and need to be handled with love, kindness and affection. I spoke to the little boy about what he could do to help his mum look after the puppies and to the mother about only allowing her children to spend time with her pets under supervision. I like to think I made a difference and that perhaps the little boy will start to treat animals with more respect in the future. Maybe nothing I said meant anything to them, but if I believed that then I may as well give up.

By the end of my shift, the male puppy had perked up a little and had managed to take some puppy milk from a syringe. It would be a long night shift for the night nurses who would need to feed them every few hours and monitor them both closely for any deterioration. At least they were in the best place now and, with any luck, if they made it through the night, they could be discharged back home to the mother dog in the next few days. She must be missing them. I put my hand on the glass of the incubator where they had been placed for warmth and watched them for a few moments, snuggled up together. It's the innocence of animals that I love, but it's also what makes it so utterly heartbreaking when they are purposefully harmed by humans who should know better. I sighed and blew them each a little kiss goodnight. I see cruelty and suffering all the time, but I know I mustn't dwell on it, both for the sake of my career and my own mental health. I have to continue to give the best I can to each animal that comes through the door.

As I walked to the tube, I reminded myself that I see a skewed population of animals in my line of work. Animal welfare over time has actually improved considerably in the UK with increased lifespans for our domesticated pets, decreased inequality and better laws on prevention of cruelty. Yes, it could still be better and there will always be sad cases like this one, but thankfully most dog owners love and cherish their pets and would be horrified at the thought of them coming to any harm.

8 MAY 2015

Crazy-but-lovely neighbour just messaged to say she's on holiday in Cornwall and a seagull has landed on her car bonnet and won't move, even when she drove the car (slowly) to the shops. She's struggling to see the road ahead, what should she do?

I messaged back a series of suggestions including beeping the horn and manually removing the bird and placing it somewhere safe. I waited in anticipation for a reply. A few moments later my phone beeped. *OK, the bird has flown away now, but a stray dog is following me to the shops and doesn't seem to have an owner. She's really sweet and seems kind of lonely. Can I keep her?*

12 MAY 2015

A client refused euthanasia for his terminally sick pet today. This happens often and is my least favourite clinical situation to deal with. Rex, a fourteen-year-old long-haired cat, came in for investigations into his dramatic weight loss. Mr Ham was guarded and defensive when we discussed Rex's condition. Rex was emaciated with bones jutting out everywhere. His black fur, once soft and fluffy, had coalesced into large matts all over his body with flakes of dandruff collecting around the base of each dreadlock. His nails were overgrown and brittle, some curling around into the fleshy parts of his pads. He had lost fifty per cent of his body weight in three months. He was dehydrated and weak, lying on the table in front of me with sunken eyes and a vacant, disconnected expression. I could tell that in his prime he would have been a mighty creature, prowling the neighbourhood and putting the feline world to rights. But some time ago he had fallen from his position of top cat and succumbed to old age and illness. The cat I saw in front of me now was a broken one.

Mr Ham reported complete lack of appetite for the last week and daily vomiting. In an elderly cat this history, together with the clinical picture, pointed towards something sinister going on. We discussed euthanasia, but I could tell that Mr Ham was not ready to have this conversation. He shot me down immediately and told me it was not an option.

'Listen, you are meant to be a doctor. Just tell me what's wrong with my cat and fix him,' he said, through gritted teeth.

I reminded myself that he was upset, worried and fearful for his furry friend of fourteen years and tried not to let his slightly aggressive manner and large frame standing over me intimidate me.

'Mr Ham, we will do some tests on Rex, but we may not find anything, and it may not change our treatment options or outcome,' I explained as calmly as possible.

I admitted Rex to the hospital and performed blood tests to check for diabetes and thyroid problems and to assess his internal organs. Nothing. I did a scan of his abdomen and took X-rays of his chest and abdomen. Nothing. I spent half a morning trying, and failing, to find out what was causing his symptoms. As you read this, many vets all over the country will be experiencing a similar scenario. It's a familiar one to us. Science only gets you so far, and we lack the many tools in our veterinary practices that human medicine has such as CT or MRI. These are mostly only available in referral practices. I reluctantly picked up the phone and called Mr Ham. I explained the tests we had done and the results. We had ruled several things out, but essentially we still had no answers. I advised him that Rex could well have a brain tumour or other cancer in his body that we had been unable to find. I offered referral to another practice or to a specialist if Mr Ham wished to get another opinion. I explained that as a charity we had done all we could but regardless of the underlying cause, the fact remained that Rex was a terribly sick boy and without any intervention would probably die in the coming days or weeks.

Mr Ham was furious. 'Let me get this straight. You did all those tests and still have no clue what his problem is? How can you call yourself a professional and yet you have no idea what is wrong? You say X-rays don't always find the problem, so why do you bother using them? You scanned all his organs, you're saying you found nothing and yet you want me to kill my own cat. Do you even know what you're doing?! If I don't know what's wrong with him then I'm not putting him down, no way. I'm coming to collect him this afternoon!'

After a twenty-minute cyclical conversation during which Mr Ham became increasingly irate despite my best efforts to calm him, he eventually hung up, claiming I just wanted to kill his cat and he wasn't 'having it'. I sighed, felt the supportive pat of my vet colleague Lucy on my shoulder and we exchanged a look of resigned understanding. I looked down at Rex sitting next to me.

'Sorry, old fella,' I told him.

He raised his eyes to meet mine without lifting his head from the basket.

'I can see you've had enough. I tried.'

I took a few deep breaths and tried to calm my heart rate down before returning him to his kennel and fetching the next patient.

I discharged Rex later this afternoon. If a cat at the end of its life doesn't want to eat through illness, nothing you can do will make it eat. I was pretty sure that Rex would waste away at home and eventually slip into a coma, dying slowly from dehydration and starvation and from the cancer that I suspected was eating him from the inside, without even the option of opioid painkillers and sedatives that humans have access to at the end. My professional duty involves recommending what is best for the animals under my care, even if this means being used as a punching bag by clients like Mr Ham who do not like what I have to say. Sadly, many owners confuse vets' trained and professional recommendations with a desire to terminate animals lives unnecessarily and this couldn't be further from the truth. I think part of the issue is that owners understandably can't face making that final decision. They see putting their pet to sleep as a choice to end their pet's life, whereas in very sick animals the decision has often already been made for them. Euthanasia merely prevents further suffering and allows terminal patients a dignified and painless end.

In recognition of the fact that making a euthanasia decision can be one of the most difficult decisions people make in their lives, many veterinary practices are now offering owners quality-of-life questionnaires to complete on their pets' behalf. The quality of animals' (and humans') lives are not defined by one aspect but rather by a combination of their overall physical and mental well-being. Quality-of-life questionnaires can help owners to assess whether their pet is experiencing more 'bad' days than 'good' by answering questions about their pain levels, whether they are struggling to get around, their general behaviour and their appetite. As vets, we only see pets for a short snippet of time in our consulting room, during which they may behave very differently to how they behave in their home environment. But on the flip side, vets have a medical qualification and often years of experience of treating animals in addition to the objectivity required to assess a pet's general well-being. This is why the decision of when to let a pet go should ideally always be made together by an owner and their vet.

Euthanasia is certainly a complex and divisive topic. It's true that I have become much more numb to it as a concept after many years of doing the job. But it's also true that I have seen more suffering over these years than you can imagine. A client once said to me that it is better to put a pet to sleep a month too early than a minute too late. I think many people who have seen their loved ones suffer, both human and animal, would agree with this. I certainly do. Leaving aside the even more controversial issue of human euthanasia, which is illegal in any form in the UK, I deeply empathise with the sadness and difficulty that comes with choosing to terminate the life of your most treasured pet, friend and furry family member. I have been through that turmoil myself before with Snowy and the pain of saying goodbye and grief that followed was akin to losing a relative for me. When I put myself in my clients' shoes, imagining that Rex was Bea, and that a vet was telling me to put her to sleep without knowing what was wrong with her, I can see why clients like Mr Ham become angry and dissatisfied. But if Bea's health deteriorated and she was wasting away in front of my eyes, all the characteristics that make her the wonderful nutty cat I know and love being stolen from her one by one through illness, I like to think I would have the strength to put her first. As one of my colleagues said to me recently, 'they're here for a good time not a long time'. The questions of 'why' and 'how' are sometimes just academic. It may make us feel better to know, but it doesn't prevent suffering or delay the inevitable.

15 MAY 2015

One of the receptionists just came to tell me that Mr Ham called to let us know that Rex died at home last night. I dread to think what kind of death he endured but at least he isn't suffering anymore. Small mercies.

19 MAY 2015

Me: Have you considered getting Jimmy Chew castrated?

Mrs Montebello: Oh no, he definitely doesn't need to be. [Jimmy Chew gives me a beady eye of Pomeranian mistrust and curls a lip exposing his rotten brown teeth, just to remind me who is boss.]

Me: OK, do you mind me asking why you feel that way?

Mrs Montebello: He has Peppa Pig and she keeps him very happy.

Me: I see . . . [Attempts to withhold laughter and maintain a professional exterior.]

Mrs Montebello: Yes, his wonderful Peppa piggy toy. That's all he needs. He humps her all the time. Sometimes I struggle to separate him from his little piggy. They love each other.

I will never look at Peppa Pig the same way again. Little minx.

25 MAY 2015

For the first time in a long time, maybe ever, I was given a present by a client today. I came home and proudly displayed it on the kitchen counter for James and Bea to see. Bea approached cautiously and gave it an unimpressed sniff. It's not every day you get a box of Special K cereal bars but today was the day. Only ninety calories per bar! I shall savour each and every mouthful.

26 MAY 2015

The little puppies with the head trauma came back in to see me today. The whole family seemed very upbeat and had all been helping out with the puppies' feeding and general care. They brought the mother dog to see me as well, a cute happy two-year-old Jack Russell cross-breed, and we booked her in to have her spayed to prevent any more unwanted litters. The little boy puppy was jumping about and had made a full recovery. I felt so happy I wanted to jump up and down with him. His entire face was covered in brown muck where he had face-planted into a bowl of mushy puppy food, which simply added to his cheeky enthusiastic charm. The owner has luckily found homes for both puppies and they will soon be going off to start a new life. I gave them a cuddle goodbye and made a little prayer to the canine gods that it would be a good one.

27 MAY 2015

Crazy-but-lovely neighbour just texted. She has found a group of
hens that need saving, could we find a way to adopt them all and
keep them in our gardens? There are only thirty of them. She
attached a photo of one called Gemma, the 'caged-hen survivor'
with the description 'I was used to lay eggs and lived in hell, until
I was rescued'. An image of all the chickens in the animation film
Chicken Run marching to their deathbeds when the owners of
their farm decided to move from selling eggs to selling chicken pot
pies sprang to mind. Gemma's little face did look decidedly traumatised for a hen and for a moment I actually considered the
possibility of trying to rehouse thirty hens in my six-foot-long
city garden. I then imagined the even more traumatised look on
James's face when I tried to explain the situation to him and
thought better of it. Plus, I suspect poor Gemma's days would be
numbered once Bea caught sight of her.

28 MAY 2015

Patients come and go and many of them fade into an abyss of
spays, castrations, wounds, dentals, X-rays, skin disease and diarrhoea. Today was different. Today I said goodbye to a friend. Two
weeks ago a stray dog whom we called Pinky (because of her
white fur and pink skin, and pink little nose like a piglet) found
her way to us. Like many stray dogs brought in, she had pendulous milky teats and there was almost certainly a litter of puppies
somewhere nearby missing their mummy. Pinky was a skinny girl,
tall and leggy with a short nose and floppy ears. She looked like a
white Labrador crossed with a Staffie, with a smidgen of Boxer in
there too. She was extremely gentle, cuddly and playful, and often
spent time during her stay with us in the offices keeping members
of staff company. She had abundant energy and loved to climb (all
28kg of her) on to your lap for cuddles. She clearly could not
believe her luck to have found herself in a warm, dry environment

with food and love on tap. Pinky had skin disease, as many white-haired Staffies do, but was otherwise healthy, and I found myself sneaking up to her kennel to spend a bit of time with her in my breaks. Little by little, she crept into my heart. Sometimes, for no particular reason, you just click with an animal. Anyone who has ever owned or cared for a dog will understand immediately what I mean. They suit you, and you suit them. You become buddies. You understand one another.

When Pinky arrived at the hospital, we were legally obliged to inform the local authority that she was under our care, as we do with all stray dogs. Today, the police dog legislation officer came to assess her. After a few measurements I was told she had been deemed 'Pit Bull Terrier type' and needed to be euthanised under Section 1 of the Dangerous Dogs' Act. Stray dogs who are classified as Section 1 sadly cannot be rehomed by law. All rehoming charities including PWH are legally obliged to euthanise them regardless of whether we believe a dog can be safely and happily rehomed. The Act was introduced in 1991 in response to several serious injuries and deaths resulting from dog attacks. It is considered by many, me included, to have been a rushed and poorly considered piece of legislation. It has been criticised as ineffectual because its mandate is limited to four banned breeds – Pit Bull Terrier, Japanese Tosa, Dogo Argentino and Fila Brasileiro – rather than concentrating on the behaviour of the dogs in question. There is absolutely no evidence to suggest that these four breeds are more likely to show aggression than any other dog. Furthermore, we don't actually have genetic testing available in the UK to definitively prove that a dog belongs to a certain breed. The current decision-making process is based purely on the measurements of a dog's body conformation, a process that clearly has a huge potential for error.

My years in charity practice have taught me that any dog can show aggression if it is incorrectly trained or badly treated. Indeed, since the legislation was introduced, the number of human hospital admissions for injuries caused by dogs is at its highest. According to figures from the Health and Social Care Information Centre, between March 2005 and February 2015, dog bites in England requiring medical attention increased by 76%, highlighting the fact that the law does not help to protect people from dog-related incidents. Sadly, not only does it fail to protect members of the public but it also punishes many healthy good-natured dogs that are euthanised every year, not because they have behaved in any way aggressively or inappropriately, but because their measurements are considered breed 'type'. To me, and many members of the veterinary community, it seems completely absurd that we are making decisions about dogs' futures based on their looks alone.

Ironically, at this very moment there are thousands of aggressive dogs around the country who are lucky enough to have loving homes or have people rallying to save them; Chihuahuas who are too aggressive even to muzzle when they come to the vets; Jack Russells who bark at you with intent and you know would most likely rip your hand off if the owner let go of their lead; Collies and even so-called family-friendly Labradors that have to be muzzled in public because they are intolerant of other dogs or people, particularly children. Meanwhile, dogs who have committed no such acts are unjustifiably handed an automatic death sentence because they have the wrong body measurements despite a docile, calm and loving nature. What a pointless and unnecessary waste of life.*

*There has been widespread campaigning, including the dedicated 'SaveABulls' campaign set up by two veterinary nurses, to amend the Dangerous Dogs Act so that it is no longer breed specific. The Parliamentary Select Committee (EFRA) that scrutinises the work of DEFRA finally launched an inquiry into the Act in 2018. 'The report following the inquiry indicated that the focus on Breed Specific Legislation is misguided and that the Government's arguments in favour of maintaining Breed Specific Legislation are not substantiated by robust evidence. It recommended that to avoid imposing an

Esther held Pinky for me while I placed a catheter in her leg. She didn't even struggle. She trusted us. I fed her dog treats and fresh chicken. I asked her for her paw and she gave me each one in turn and I rewarded her with a handful of chocolate and grapes because she loved them and it didn't matter anymore that they are toxic to dogs. I kissed the top of her soft head and hugged her goodbye. I whispered into her ear that I was sorry. And then I administered an overdose of pentobarbitone and she passed away in my arms.

Today was a bad day.

29 MAY 2015

One of my favourite clients, Mr Johnson, came to see me today. I've known him for many years now, since my early days working as a new graduate at PWH. He has autism and lives alone with his two sixteen-year-old cats, Alfred and Rose, whom he adores. He is a lovely, gentle man and an extremely dedicated owner. He rescued Alfred and Rose from a PWH rehoming centre eleven years ago. He listens to every piece of advice we give him, administers every treatment with precision and care, attends every appointment on time and leaves regular contributions towards the cost of his cats' treatment. He thanks us every time he visits, which means an awful lot, and we thank him in return for coming to see us and for taking such good care of his pets.

Today he brought Alfred in for a general check-up. Alfred has dodgy kidneys but is otherwise doing pretty well for his age. Mr Johnson has an endearing tendency to repeat his cats' names with every sentence he says throughout the consultation. We chatted as

---

unnecessary death sentence on good-tempered animals, the ban on transferring Section 1 dogs to new owners should be removed immediately if the animal has been behaviourally assessed and found to be safe. Frustratingly, to date the Dangerous Dogs Act and breed specific legislation remains unchanged.

we weighed Alfred, checked his blood pressure, and made a plan for his continued care. We spoke about the weather and how Mr Johnson keeps the cats inside when it's raining in case they catch a cold. He told me he had been staying up late to tempt Arthur to eat as he is picky with his food and both cats like to have their back stroked while they are eating. He loves nothing more than to sit watching television in the evening with his cats, one (Arthur) on his lap and the other (Rose) by his feet. She's never been a lap cat, he explained.

After he left, I thought about how some days at PWH have felt like walking through treacle recently. There have been so many lovely clients, but the ones that have stood out have sadly been the welfare cases, the abusive clients and the clients who have left it too long before seeking veterinary treatment for their sick pets. Seeing Mr Johnson today was the tonic I needed. He is an embodiment of what PWH is here for, and why I still feel proud to work for them. There is no way Mr Johnson, or others like him, would be able to afford private veterinary fees and he so deserves the support and help that charity veterinary services provide. And it is certainly not a one-way street. Being surrounded by other animal lovers and dedicated, caring owners is heart-warming for vets, and helps to soften the blow of the Pinkys, the Zias, the Ebonys and the Winnies. Mr Johnson and the many other clients like him provide me with a regular reminder of how wonderful this job can be and how privileged I am to be doing it.

Part 4

SUMMER

1 JUNE 2015
PARASITES FOR DUMMIES

How to remove a tick:
Purchase tick remover from Amazon for £2.99. Remove tick.

How not to remove a tick:
Burn it off with a cigarette.
Get your other dog to bite it off.
Spray it with Dettol.
Drown it by bathing your pet for one hour every day (no more, no less).
Twirl it around and around until it becomes too dizzy to cling on.

2 JUNE 2015

Just had the pleasure of seeing Ms Bosewood and her cat Spice and Pit Bull Peppa. Both animals have fleas – one of many parasite consultations I will be seeing now summer has arrived. I knew they had fleas not just because of the black creepy crawlies I observed running through their fur, or the flea dirt and itchy scabs on their skin, but because Ms Bosewood herself has succumbed to some itchy flea bites.* As vets, we become used to clients

---

*Flea dirt is the black debris you can see on an animal's fur when they have a flea infestation. Delightfully, it is actually flea poo which the disgusting creatures will eat in addition to feeding off your pet's blood to prolong their lifecycle. People say if the world ended only cockroaches would survive. I disagree – in a contest of durability, fleas would win every time.

showing us bits of their bodies, asking what we think of a rash or infected bite or whether something is caused by mange or ringworm or bedbugs. Generally, however, the lesions are on people's arms or necks or ankles, or at worst their cleavage. Not the case for Ms Bosewood. Her bites were located on her upper thighs and buttocks.

Unfortunately, she also happened to be wearing skinny jeans, making access to her thigh bites difficult. So down came her jeans. As she started to unbuckle her belt and unzip them, much to the dismay of her teenage daughter, I protested and explained that examining the pets was enough evidence for me and seeing her bites really was unnecessary. She insisted, however, and luckily was wearing a thong so the view of her buttock bites was pretty easy once her trousers were down at her ankles. As she bent over to flash her white bum cheeks at me I averted my eyes and in that uncomfortable prudish British way started babbling rapidly about the lifecycle of the flea and avoiding eye contact with her teenage daughter at all costs, who was by now hiding in the corner of the room frantically texting on her mobile phone. Something along the lines of, *Send help: Mother's gone loco*, I should imagine. Just at this moment one of my male colleagues entered the room. I jumped up and practically cartwheeled across the room to the door, closing it in his confused face in an attempt to preserve Ms Bosewood's dignity.

Peppa, who had become rather excited by all the commotion, did a little puddle of excitement wee and then proceeded to run rings around Ms Bosewood's skinny-jean-clad ankles, tethering her legs together further with the extendable lead. After some potato-sack-race-style jumping and frantic forearm circling, Ms Bosewood lost her balance and toppled to the ground, landing bottom down in the puddle of Peppa's urine. Thankfully, I had a large towel to hand and thrust it over Ms Bosewood, attempting to mop up the urine around her while carefully avoiding groping her thighs. As she stood up I got a far closer look at the spots on her bottom than I had anticipated. Turns out they weren't flea bites after all, but whiteheads.

'Maybe pop to the GP about those spots and get them checked, in case they need some treatment,' I said. 'And perhaps wear a skirt to your appointment?'

3 JUNE 2015

Me: Is he a friendly boy? [This is vet talk for 'will he savage my face if I examine him?']

Owner: Oh yes, always.

Me: It's just he's curling his lip up like he's a bit cross. [Steps back from Prince the Chihuahua who is staring at me like he wants to take me down.]

Owner: No, he always does that. Really, he would never bite.

Me: It might be worth putting a muzzle on him just in case, especially as I'm about to empty his anal glands.

Owner: [Looking disgruntled.] No, he doesn't need one. I'll hold him. No other vets have ever had to muzzle him.

Me: Nonetheless, he's holding his ears back and growling at me, best to be safe.

Owner: I'm not happy about this. Why can't we see that nice man we saw last time.

Me: [Checks computer, previous vet has written 'CARE: WILL BITE' following his clinical examination notes.] I'm afraid he's not available so if you want me to empty his anal glands today I really would prefer to muzzle him.

Owner: Fine. But before you do that can you check his teeth?

Me: . . .

4 JUNE 2015

I've been working with a vet student the last two weeks whom I have become rather fond of. She's one of the good ones – not that we see many 'bad' ones. The calibre of new graduate vets coming out of UK veterinary schools is exceptional. Their knowledge and confidence is often inspiring, despite their lack of experience.

Leila has been observing me consulting and scrubbing into my surgeries and I like to think she's had a memorable and useful experience spending time with me. I have always loved teaching. Possibly inspired by my mother, sister, James and numerous friends who have all been school teachers at various stages, I think it's a wholly worthwhile and deeply important job. Despite its bureaucracy and endless paperwork, it's certainly a profession I would have considered had veterinary medicine not worked out for me.

I remember being fourteen years old and seeing practice at a veterinary charity near where I grew up. It was a school placement and I had been really excited about it. The senior vet there was examining a lump on a dog's side. He told me to have a feel of the lump, which I did, gently. He laughed unpleasantly at me and then said rather callously, 'I can tell you'll never be a vet. That's not how you feel a lump. You have to actually get your hands around it and *feeeeel* it. Not that useless soft little prod you're doing.' And then, with a smirk, he moved on with his examination. The nurse in the room with us gave me a withered look of sympathy. He thought I would never be a vet. It was a quick and flippant remark that he will have forgotten instantly, but it hit me round the face like a sharp slap. I had admired him, despite his rough bedside manner, because he was a veterinary surgeon. Someone to be trusted. His comments had damaged my fragile teenage self-confidence.

Of course, nearly twenty years later, I have the wisdom to real- ise that this particular vet was just an unpleasant man who, in hindsight, didn't treat his staff very kindly let alone the school students he came across. I have since encountered many more men and women like him at vet school and in general life who feel that using humiliation and derogatory terminology rather than encouragement and praise are respectable ways to teach. I was secretly delighted to discover when I bumped into one of the nurses at that practice after I graduated that the senior vet in question had been dismissed for poor professional conduct a few years after I met him. But the experience made me realise that the words and tone influential members of society use to address those who are learning from them can make an enormous difference to their well-being and self-belief. It's not easy being a vet student, being sent to a new practice every week, trying your best to prove yourself again and again. In fact, it's exhausting. So now when I spend time with students, I try not to get frustrated when I am in a hurry and they are standing in my way, or asking questions at an inopportune moment. I offer them my seat in theatre, or when I am consulting if I'm not using it because, frankly, standing still 'observing' for ten hours a day is hard on the legs. And if it means Leila goes home feeling excited about what's to come rather than dreading each day she spends with me, then it's worth the extra effort.

5 JUNE 2015

Leila seemed a little upset this morning when she arrived at the hospital. I asked her if anything was wrong, and she replied tearfully that one of her vet friends at university had committed suicide yesterday. I felt terribly sad for her, but it was not, alas, the first time I had come across this scenario within the veterinary profession. Sadly, mental health problems are rife among vets. In the seventies and eighties, veterinary medicine was in fact the occupation in the UK with the highest suicide rate for both men and women. More recently, in a study conducted between 2001 and 2005 comparing different professions across Britain, vets were still third in line for suicide among women, behind sports players and artists. Compared to the general population, male vets are three times more likely, and female vets four to six times more likely, to die by suicide in the UK. In America, studies have also shown disproportionately high rates of depression and anxiety among vets, with a suicide rate up to four times higher than the general population. The first mental health survey of US vets, published in March 2015, showed that one in six vets have considered suicide since graduating. Meanwhile, the *Canadian Veterinary Journal* published findings in January 2015 from a 'wellness' survey, which found that 19% of Canadian vets had considered suicide and 9% had attempted it, with 49% of those claiming they were still at risk of a repeat episode.

During the course of the day, Leila's experience of losing her friend kept reminding me of a vet I had worked with when I was a student and he was newly qualified. I was in deepest darkest Devon seeing practice at a farm animal vets in my final year with my friend Katharine. I had been working with Owen, a fresh-faced, blue-eyed Irish man in his mid-twenties, for most of the week. He was softly spoken, cute looking and very humble. We had finished a day of calls and he turned to me before I got out of the car. I gazed into his big blue eyes.

'Charlotte . . .' he said in his lovely Irish accent.

'Yes?' I swooned.

'You've got a bit of shit on your face.'

Oh crap. I felt my face turn a shade of beetroot and quickly started rubbing at the cow poo which soon turned into more of a faecal face mask.

'I'll contact you and your pal Katharine tonight if we have any emergencies come in,' he said.

I thanked him and then made a dash to the loo to sort out my face. Later that evening we did indeed receive a call from Owen to say that he was headed out to an emergency bovine C-section, if we wanted to join him. He gave us the postcode and off we went into the night. Of course, we got hopelessly lost after our TomTom directed us into a hedge. Finally, we found the farm, changed into our overalls and wellies, and fumbled our way across the fields and down to the cowshed in the darkness. As we approached I could see the dull beam of his car headlights shining into the barn. This appeared to be the only light available. I squinted to see what was happening. There was complete silence and I couldn't see any movement either. As we walked the last few metres I suddenly made out the scene in front of me and a feeling of dread took hold.

The fully grown 800kg Belgian Blue cow was lying dead on the floor. There was blood everywhere. She had a large caesarean cut to her side exposing her organs beneath. A metre away lay her calf who was also dead. I glanced up in horror and saw the farmer leaning against the edge of the barn shaking his head. His face was grief-stricken. Anyone who thinks that farmers see their livestock as only commodities is gravely mistaken. Many of the cattle farmers I've met over the years have cared deeply about their cows. Yes, it is a working relationship and they are ultimately being used as part of a business model and, as such, a degree of rational thought and emotional separation must be applied. But the majority of farmers would never wish to see harm to their animals and they try to protect them and provide them with the best quality of life they can. To see one of them die in front of your eyes is a crushing experience, whatever the circumstances.

After a few moments my attention was drawn away from the farmer to the corner of the barn where Owen sat in his waterproofs, covered head to toe in blood, with his head in his hands. Katharine and I looked at each other in shock. Neither of us dared to speak or move a muscle. The silence was eventually broken after what seemed an impossible length of time by the farmer making a call to his herdsman.

'Yes, she's dead too . . . No . . . About a grand . . . I know . . . absolutely awful . . .'

I could hear him talking in hushed tones.

We finally broke our trance and approached Owen. 'Are you OK?' I asked him tentatively.

'There wasn't enough light. I couldn't find the source of the bleeding . . . I couldn't save them. I tried . . .' He trailed off.

'Can we do anything?' Katharine asked.

'No, no. It's best you go home, girls. I'm sorry you had to see this,' he replied.

I noticed his hands, covered in blood and straw, were trembling. We helped him to clean up the worst of the blood and then, not wishing to get in the way, headed back to our car in silence.

The next morning we arrived at the practice and the general mood was melancholic. We had another week still to go but Owen didn't appear for the remainder of our time there. I have no idea what happened to him but I have never forgotten the broken look on his face sitting in that gloomy barn. Many times I've wondered since how the events of that night impacted his self-confidence and the rest of his career. Whether he ever fully recovered. He seemed to me to be a prime example of how things can go drastically wrong for vets and why, unless we have the right support network, many vets end up suffering bouts of anxiety or depression or, at the very least, feelings of inadequacy throughout our careers.

The disproportionately poor mental health and high suicide rates among vets are rarely talked about outside the profession. When I've mentioned the issue to friends who are not vets, they are always shocked and almost always go on to ask whether it's because of the emotional stress of euthanising animals. I can understand why they might think this, but for the majority of vets, euthanasia is actually seen as a way of relieving suffering rather than a burden. Perhaps there is an argument that regular euthanasia normalises death as a solution to problems for vets. But I suspect that is oversimplifying the matter and the cause is actually multimodal. Yes, we see euthanasia as a solution to unsolvable problems and this thought process could be transferred over to humans. But it's not vets' perceptions of death as a pragmatic way out that is most alarming, it is how frequently they reach the point where it even becomes a consideration.

Vets often have 'type A' perfectionist personalities, characterised by excessive ambition, dedication, drive and organisation – all traits that make us good at what we do. But there is a dark side to our perfectionism and compassion. Frequent university exams and the pressures of passing them followed by long antisocial hours and high stress levels within the profession can cause havoc with even the most robust person's mental health. Then there is the financial burden many vets face of paying back unimaginable levels of debt post university, with relatively modest salaries compared to other medical practitioners and considering the hours worked and level of responsibility we have. In the years since I graduated, a further stress factor has now been added to the mix, and that is social media. A vet friend of mine saw a client recently who filmed their consultation in which they discussed neutering in order to name and shame her on social media because the client found the topic unsavoury and did not wish to neuter her pet. My friend had merely been concerned about the pet's well-being, but soon found herself at the heart of an angry online debate. Social media has developed in the last decade from a useful tool used to advertise practice policies and opening hours, spread the word about animal welfare and reach out to new clients, to a weapon used by disgruntled owners who wish to make their feelings publicly known, however hurtful or slanderous they might be. I am absolutely pro freedom of speech, but vets all over the world are sadly being persecuted online by people who were not even involved in the issues raised and, unsurprisingly, it is starting to take its toll.

Finally, and perhaps most worryingly, vets have easy access to dangerous drugs combined with the knowledge of how to use them. If or when vets have suicidal thoughts and decide to act on them, they are likely to be successful. I can understand when grouping all these factors together why our small body of people are so vulnerable, and frankly I don't know what the solution is. Contacting the Samaritans may be a good place to start. They are available 24/7 to offer support, practical advice and information to anyone in need. In America, a confidential support group called Vets4Vets has been created, offering vets one-to-one crisis management and mindfulness meditation sessions. Similarly, a charity called Vetlife was set up in the UK with the aim of helping vets in moments of crisis. Formed a century ago under the name 'The Veterinary Benevolence Society', Vetlife opened a helpline in the eighties. They are a well-used service, receiving over a thousand new contacts per year from the 20,000 practising vets in the UK. So each year a minimum of one in twenty vets reaches crisis point, and that is only counting the ones who reach out for help.* Surely there must be a way to reduce the stress burden and prevent burn-out before it gets to that stage?

The newly established veterinary mentor schemes across the UK should hopefully reduce the number of vets becoming unhappy due to lack of adequate support early on in their careers. Vetlife has been encouraging vets to leave the veterinary profession entirely if they find that it is impacting on their mental health. This seems like sound advice when considering the high suicide rate we are faced with. Many of my friends whom I graduated alongside years ago have now sadly abandoned veterinary medicine. They have gone on to have wonderful and fulfilling lives in other areas including teaching, becoming parents, working for the government, becoming lawyers and working for drug companies. They work fewer and more regular hours, in some cases are better paid, and in almost all cases are happier and less stressed. They were all really great vets and it is a loss to the profession, but as special as it can be, it can also be a disheartening and emotionally draining job. Reportedly up to 40% of UK vets leave the job within the first five years of graduating. A national veterinary

---

*Flash forward to 2020 and this figure has more than doubled, with over 2,500 new Vetlife contacts. In 2017, a well regarded vet who was a trustee of Vetlife and co-founder of a veterinary support group called Veterinary Voices UK, tragically commited suicide. After hearing about this, a clothing company called Smith-Webb, who support mental health and anti-bullying charities, agreed to donate a proportion of sales of their jumpers, emblazoned with the words 'Be Kind', to Vetlife in her memory. Vets all over the country have now started to wear 'Be Kind' jumpers to highlight the importance of supporting and nurturing one another.

recruitment crisis has been declared following the outflow of vets and veterinary nurses to other professions.[*]

In my experience, vets have an instinctual desire to hide their emotions and pretend everything is 'fine' at all times. Perhaps this is in part due to the fact that, despite their high prevalence among vets, mental health issues are still taboo in many practices. Continuing to expose and normalise mental illness nationally and within the profession seems imperative. In addition, we need to break away from the current and unsustainable trend of working 12 to 14 hours per day in an emotional and unpredictable environment with mounting client expectation for an immediate service, or instant fix for their pet's ailments. Vets must be encouraged to accept their feelings rather than hiding them or denying the warning signs in order to prevent catastrophic events from occurring before it's too late. We must learn to let go and stop punishing ourselves when a treatment option eludes us or a patient under our care dies despite our best efforts. Establishing a support network and promoting kindness and openness within the workplace are surely fundamental if we are to face this problem as a profession rather than shying away from it as we have done, shamefully, for over half a century.

I went to talk to a group of A Level students about becoming vets last year and I had to reign in my desire to warn them about the potential strains and pitfalls of the career. I forced myself to put a smile on my face and discuss all the positive aspects of the job, of which there are of course many. But since that day I have started to wonder whether potential student vets do need to be

---

[*]Brexit has predictably compounded this issue. The Institute of Employment Studies found that 18% of EU vets working in the UK in 2018 were actively looking to leave, while 32% were considering leaving, and 40% were more likely to leave. With Brexit details still unclear in 2020, if stricter immigration rules are brought into law, I am left wondering how the industry would cope if it were to lose 50% of its workforce. We may need to rapidly consider what can be done to encourage more people to take up the profession in the UK should we lose our valuable European veterinarians.

educated about compassion fatigue before beginning a career in veterinary medicine. Perhaps a greater awareness at that early stage and an altered mindset that it is perfectly normal to reach out for help, and it does not mean you have failed in any way, is just what the profession needs. I am very aware that I've been lucky. I landed myself a job soon after graduation that I loved and always had colleagues who've helped me through the dark days. But without their support, and that of my family, I think I would ultimately have followed suit and become yet another vet who didn't want to be a vet anymore.

I went out in my lunch break today and bought Leila some dough-nuts. Sometimes it's the small things in life that make a difference, and sugary balls of carbohydrate seemed as good a consolation as any. She will get through it, and will go on to graduate and become a wonderful vet, I'm sure. But I can't help but worry that this is simply the first of many bumps she will feel along the unpredictable road of veterinary medicine.

8 JUNE 2015

An email just arrived in my inbox inviting me to attend the following course: *Will you be sued in 2015? Top tips for avoiding an employment tribunal.*

How depressing. How about I summarise it in a couple of sentences to save eight hours of my time and £300 of my money:

Vets – don't do anything to a client's animal that you wouldn't do to your own.

Clients – remember we're only human and we can't always save your pet, no matter how hard we try. And, believe me, we try.

9 JUNE 2015

Just finished a Friday afternoon enema double whammy. A constipated cat followed by a Bulldog that had eaten his own body
weight in lamb bones.

Please, I beg of you, do not feed bones to your dog. Contrary to
popular belief, they are not a lovely 'treat' for your pet. They will
shred your dog's intestine in a similar manner to a razor blade,
and can cause severe vomiting, diarrhoea, ulceration, constipa-
tion, blood loss and even death. Give them Schmackos instead
(the dog version of Dreamies) – far yummier and less lethal.

Off to my friend's wedding later this evening for a weekend of celebrating and I appear to have committed the ultimate veterinary sin
and forgotten to double glove. Nothing quite says 'lifetime commitment' like the foul rotten stench of faeces on one of your wedding
guests. Still, at least I will get a seat on the tube home. Silver linings
and all that.

10 JUNE 2015

An axolotl was abandoned on the doorstep of the hospital over
the weekend. An axo-what-ol? I hear you cry. Wikipedia informed
me that an axolotl, also known as a Mexican salamander or
Mexican 'walking fish', is a salamander that is closely related to
the tiger salamander. They certainly should not be confused
with waterdogs, the larval stage of the closely related tiger salamanders, or mudpuppies which are fully aquatic salamanders. Eh?
Unsurprisingly, none of this information helped me as my knowledge of salamanders is equal to that of axolotls: non-existent.

I made a quick call to my amphibian-obsessed nephew to find
out what it actually was, and what I should do with it. Luckily, he
surpassed my expectations and not only knew what diet they
should be fed, but also helped me to understand why the poor fella
was missing his characteristic pink feathery gills. It would seem he

had not been kept in the right environment to allow him to flourish and hopefully once that's corrected he will go on to live a happy life. I've called him Axel Rose, of course. He resembles a swimming version of Falcor, the white scaly flying dogfish from *The Labyrinth*, for anyone who loves eighties' movies as much as I do. He's quite cute, all things considered, and I thought about adopting him myself but the size of tank he would need would take up half of my living room. This is what troubles me about amphibians and reptiles being kept in captivity. So many of them are abandoned or suffer horrible illnesses because of poor husbandry or inappropriate cage size. I can't help but feel they are all better off in the wild, wandering about in the desert or rainforest in ideal temperatures for their bodies with no one fiddling about with UV lamps above their heads. Obviously, don't tell my nephew, or his lizard Spike, that I said that.

11 JUNE 2015

Today was the court case for Ruby, the lovely Staffie who came in collapsed with bad mastitis after being used as a breeding machine all those months ago. She did so well in the end. The whole hospital fell predictably in love with her, and she went to a foster home about six weeks after she first arrived. Now, six months later, she is barely recognisable from the dog that arrived all that time ago. I saw her briefly when she came in for a check-up two weeks ago. Shiny coat, wagging tail, a happy girl. She had gained 6kg in weight and looked in perfect body condition.

I felt nervous as I got dressed this morning in my smartest clothes and made my way to the court. After several hours of waiting I was ushered into the courtroom. Thankfully, Mr Kirwan pleaded guilty at the last minute, which meant I didn't need to take the stand to give my evidence. This was a big relief. I'd been up a lot in the night worrying and semi-dreaming about it, imagining being cross-examined by an angry defence lawyer with me firing back phrases from courtroom movies like, 'The truth, the truth, you can't handle the truth!' The reality was far less dramatic. I sat at the edge of the court watching the proceedings as parts of my statement were read out by the prosecuting lawyer. I made eye contact with Mr Kirwan at one point and couldn't help feeling slightly intimidated by his hard glare. The judge rounded up the case quickly and firmly, sparing Mr Kirwan a prison sentence but deeming him unfit to care for animals and banning him from doing so for a minimum of seven years. In addition, he was fined £3,000, which did not seem enough in comparison to the trauma he had inflicted on Ruby, not to mention the financial cost to PWH for six weeks' of her treatment and intensive care. I left the court watching my back, eager to disappear into the crowds before Mr Kirwan noticed me.

I was pleased overall with the result, but I wondered as I waited at the bus stop how they were going to 'police' his ban on owning animals. Working for PWH has given me quite an insight into how often animals, particularly dogs, are passed from one home to the next, and treated like commodities rather than sentient beings.*

One afternoon I examined a dog from a household from which I'd seen another dog several weeks earlier for a different condition. When the dog arrived, I could see immediately it was a different dog to the last one I had treated. It was a different size and colour, but registered under the previous dog's name and address. Unfortunately, the dog was not

*Rather alarmingly, the proposed legislation following the UK's withdrawal from the EU in 2019 will no longer incorporate the formal recognition of animal sentience. If this goes ahead it will mean that the UK no longer recognises animals as being capable of feeling joy or suffering, contrary to the extensive body of evidence which demonstrates that their conscious awareness and the richness of their experiences can, in many species, be likened to humans. This seems like a terrifying step backwards in animal welfare to me, particularly for the wild and commercially farmed animals we live alongside in Britain.

microchipped. The owner had refused to get any of his dogs chipped so I could not prove that it was a different dog. This is not an uncommon scenario in charity practice. In line with the other animal charities across the UK, we have a restriction on the number of pets we will see per household. The client that day was one of many who have multiple dogs and pass them around a variety of different addresses and there is absolutely nothing we can do about it. So the chance of Mr Kirwan having another pet under his roof at some stage in the next seven years, albeit transiently, was high.

I suppose all we can do as vets is keep chipping away trying to educate people about their duty of care, while attempting to save those animals already suffering. I couldn't help feeling a bit blue, though, thinking about the next dog that would cross Mr Kirwan's path. Maybe not today, maybe not even next year, but someday it would happen all over again. I sighed, jumped on the bus, and headed into work to start consulting.

12 JUNE 2015

Mr Hill, a gentle sweet elderly man who is hard of hearing, came in to discuss Eddie's issues with urinating today. Eddie is a ten-year-old Border Terrier with an enlarged prostate gland, which occurs commonly in older male dogs and is usually treated by castration.

Me: [Speaking very loudly despite knowing that Mr Hill can't hear me.] We need to consider getting Eddie castrated as his big prostate is making him want to wee more.
Mr Hill: [Blank face.]
Me: [Gesticulates wildly, doing my best twisting the light bulb followed by chopping the cabbage dance moves and then cupping Eddie's testicles in my hands, causing Eddie to turn around and attempt a chopping the cabbage move with his teeth on my hand.]

Mr Hill: [Blank face.]

Me: [Draws large round testicles on a piece of paper – I have never been much of an artist and on second glance these look more like Mr and Mrs Potato head from *Toy Story* – followed by a dramatic scissor motion with my hand.]

Mr Hill: [Nods and starts to smile and gives me the thumbs up.]

Either we have a mutual understanding that Eddie will soon be losing his manhood, or Mr Hill is keen to come clubbing with me after a swift game of rock/paper/scissors.

15 JUNE 2015

I chastised myself heavily over the weekend for having my work emails on my phone. I really must remove them. I arrived home on Friday after a busy day looking forward to a night of ordering pizza and relaxing in front of rubbish TV with a glass of wine. I heard a ping on my phone and stupidly found myself reading through a work email from my boss informing me that one of my clients had made an official complaint about me. Shit. Perhaps I was in need of the 'top tips for avoiding employment tribunal' course after all.

A sense of dread washed over me as I scanned the email and tried to remember the consultation and what I may have done to offend her. Despite many threats and the occasional dissatisfied client, this was the first time I had received an actual written complaint since I graduated and it hit me in the face like a hard and unexpected slap. It made itself present in my living room and lingered like a bad smell for the remainder of the evening. It wafted around me over the course of the weekend and followed me from room to room, mocking me, badgering me, refusing to let me forget that I am human and fallible and that I may have messed up. The part that stung the most was that the complaint was based around a euthanasia appointment, something I always try to approach gently and kindly. I make an enormous effort to give clients the time and patience they need at those moments just as the vet had done for me and Snowy all those years ago.

As soon as I arrived at work this morning I looked up the case and read through my clinical notes. The appointment itself had taken place over three months earlier – no wonder I had struggled to recall the details over the weekend. I must have done close to a hundred euthanasias since then. As I suspected, there was nothing that jumped out as being particularly unusual about the procedure itself, from my point of view at least, although my notes reminded me that the client, Ms Armstrong, had initially been refusing to have her eighteen-year-old Persian cat, Phoenix, put to sleep. Her complaint was based around the fact that she hadn't been ready to let him go, that in hindsight she felt Phoenix could have gone on for longer and that I should have offered her more treatment options. Sadly, Phoenix had come to see me as an emaciated, dehydrated and depressed cat who had end-stage kidney disease and had not eaten for several days. We had been treating his kidneys for some time palliatively and had had him in the hospital for stints on fluids and pain relief in the past. Several vets before me had broached the subject of euthanasia with Ms Armstrong and she hadn't been ready, but Phoenix's body had finally given up by the time he came to see me and he was, in my opinion, suffering. Both clinically and morally, the right thing to do was to let him go. The more I thought about it, the more certain I felt that I had acted in the best interests of my patient. I had discussed the option of putting him to sleep there and then, versus the other options of Ms Armstrong taking Phoenix home for a short period of time to say goodbye, or booking an appointment later that day or the next day to re-discuss the issue. Initially Ms Armstrong challenged my opinion which is completely understandable. She asked why we couldn't simply treat Phoenix with fluids and painkillers again considering they had always worked in the past. I tried to explain that Phoenix's condition had deteriorated and even if he picked up transiently on fluids, further deterioration would sadly be inevitable. I was very concerned about his absent appetite and sullen demeanour. Ms Armstrong became very quiet and stood shaking her head and stroking Phoenix while I spoke as he lay quietly on the consulting room table, sapped of energy. She occasionally interrupted me with the words, 'I just don't think I can do it.'

After our ten-minute consultation had extended to forty-five minutes, and with a waiting room full of other clients becoming agitated due to the late running of their appointments, I had finally had to encourage Ms Armstrong to make a decision about what she wanted to do. She chose to take some time in the next room to consider her options while I continued to see other patients. After half an hour more had passed, I went to see her and together – or so I had thought – we came to the decision that Phoenix would be put to sleep. I remember the euthanasia being peaceful. I remember Phoenix passing quickly as there wasn't much life left in him. I remember Ms Armstrong being sad and silent and I also remember comforting her verbally as best as I could before leaving her to spend some time with Phoenix's body. In my experience, most owners are in a conflicted state when their pet is put to sleep. It is rarely an easy or clear-cut decision. It is a time for selflessness and for prioritising a painless end for a member of your family, albeit a furry four-legged one. You desperately want to keep them alive but you don't want them to suffer, and there lies the crux of the internal conflict. What is right for them is not necessarily right for you. It was not abnormal for me to spend time persuading an owner that their pet wasn't doing well and couldn't be cured. I am as certain as I can be that if Ms Armstrong hadn't decided to put Phoenix to sleep that day then he would have passed away slowly and painfully anyway over the days, or possibly even hours, that followed.

My boss was extremely supportive about the complaint when I spoke to him during my lunch break. He showed me the three-page A4 letter of complaint that Ms Armstrong had written. Crikey, she was not a happy lady. He planned to write back to her to arrange a meeting to discuss the matter further. I explained my

version of events to him and that I felt I had behaved professionally and had not done anything that I considered negligent or
against my code of ethics. What concerned me, though, was that
I had walked away from the consultation feeling one way about it,
and the client had walked away clearly feeling very differently. I
thought long and hard about it and hypothesised what I could do
differently next time, but I struggled to see how I could change
any of the events of that day. Had my tone been in any way inappropriate, or had I rushed her or made her feel she wasn't able to
confide in me? I knew I had been telling her truths she hadn't
wanted to hear, but could I have spoken more gently or been more
aware of her dissatisfaction with the end result of the consultation? I asked myself why she hadn't said something at the time if
she wasn't happy. But I knew the answer even as the question
formed in my mind; just as grief can make people behave irration-
ally, it can also silence them. With time, she had clearly built up
feelings of regret and anger that she could finally now vocalise
and she had redirected them towards me.

I went about my job for the rest of the day with a tinge of sadness,
hyper aware of my tone and how I was expressing myself to clients. I
couldn't relax in my own skin and found my usual love of chatting to
clients had been somehow tarnished. When I got home this evening I
sat with Bea and James and flopped my head back on the sofa in
defeat. I am a people pleaser, it's part of my nature, but I was going
to have to accept that I couldn't please everyone. I knew I was lucky
as many vets receive their first complaint much sooner, and if they
are unlucky (or deserving in a minority of cases), it will go straight to
the RCVS rather than just to their practice manager. I knew that in
the weeks to come there would be letters and phone calls and I would
have to continue to defend myself and apologise to the client, despite
not fully understanding what I had done wrong. And in the meantime I would need to try and un-slump myself and continue to practise the best medicine I could without constantly looking over my
shoulder. But my confidence had been dented and, for tonight at
least, I just wanted to hide away from it all.

16 JUNE 2015

Wobble, a ten-year-old Yorkshire Terrier, came in as an emergency yesterday. His owner, Mr Pratt, had run over him with his mobility scooter. Poor Wobble was almost unconscious when he arrived, lying on one side with an oozing cut across his forehead, paddling his front legs in a swimming motion and intermittently yelping. I admitted him immediately for treatment and a quick X-ray confirmed a fractured skull. Mr Pratt was understandably beside himself.

Amazingly, less than twenty-four hours later, Wobble was sitting up yapping away when I assessed him this morning as if nothing had happened, other than a slightly odd gait and the wound on his head. Lesson learned for Mr Pratt who had let obese little Wobble down to walk on the ground following advice from a vet on weight loss. Never again will he make the same mistake. Better wobbly and alive than slim and squashed.

17 JUNE 2015

I found a note in my pigeonhole today from Ms Cruz after putting Precious to sleep last week. Precious had lasted way longer than we had thought. Clearly a combination of love and honey roasted ham is the key to longevity. It was a predictably sad and emotional goodbye when it finally came but the procedure went smoothly under the circumstances. I popped the note in my pocket without reading it and found it later when I was on the tube home. It read:

> I wanted to thank you for your kindness at the end. You were so gentle and made the trauma of it bearable. Precious was, and still is, my heartbeat. I see her everywhere. We would chat all the time. She was such a good listener! I can't bear to go out because when I get back I know she won't be there. We ate together, slept together, went on adventures together. So many memories. The games we played, the cuddles we had. Eduardo is wondering around now like a lost soul, clinging to me like a shadow. Thank goodness for

him or I would have no one left to talk to. We will come in to see you soon. Once again, thank you. The only consolation I have now is that every second of every day she knew she was loved.

With best wishes,
Ms Cristina Cruz

I finished the letter and realised I was crying in the middle of a packed, rush-hour tube carriage. The words seemed to summarise how so many owners feel after the loss of their pet, me included. That deep and unimaginable sense of loss. Seeing something move out of the corner of your eye at home, assuming it's them and then realising they aren't there anymore and that they won't ever be again. It tugged at my heartstrings. I also don't think owners realise how important their words of gratitude can be to us vets, especially in the face of an often thankless and frequently emotionally draining job. Small gestures go an awfully long way and can make an otherwise gruelling day end peacefully, despite the sadness. All humans want to feel appreciated from time to time and be reassured that they are doing a good job, and a letter from a client I adore came as a particular comfort after the euthanasia complaint I received last week.

As the tears continued to flow, I attempted to bury my face in the *Evening Standard* and found myself reading about Donald Trump, who announced yesterday that he would be running in the next presidential election. It must be a practical joke.

22 JUNE 2015

Esther brought Winnie in today for a check-up. She was worried that Winnie had never fully recovered from the last painful flare-up she had a few months ago. She potters about as usual but her limbs spasm regularly, and she chews at her back legs from time to time when the pain gets too much. She has episodes of restlessness and seems unable to readjust to normal life. Esther has been leaving her at home when she walks her other dog and so Winnie is spending a lot of her time in the house. We both agreed that her quality of life had reduced in recent months.

I examined Winnie, who growled at me and eyeballed me with her usual look of mistrust. At least that was a good sign. The day she stopped regarding me with utter contempt would be the day I would really worry.

'I'm sorry, sweetheart,' I said gently, as I prodded her spine and manipulated her sore hips. My eyes were drawn to the large scar over her right hip from her previous surgery. Memories of that innocent but terrified puppy I had met all those years ago, and images of the X-rays as more and more fractures all over her body had been identified, came flooding back to me. I felt momentary anger rise inside me. How dare a human being do this to an animal? She should still be in the prime of her life but instead she was living every day in pain because of her previous owner. I suppressed my negative thoughts and continued with my examination. When I'd finished, Winnie plopped herself down into her wonky and unique sitting position and looked up adoringly at Esther with her big Staffie grin. I suggested to Esther that she increase one of the painkillers further, to the maximum possible dose. The other drugs she was on were already at their maximum. We had exhausted many other options, including hydrotherapy and acupuncture. We made a plan for her to lose some weight as every extra pound would be additional effort on those sore limbs. We discussed short frequent walks, nothing too strenuous, and decided to give her another couple of months to see how things go. And we spoke about euthanasia when the time came. Esther discussed it with dignity and poise. She would never let Winnie suffer unnecessarily despite her own devastation at the thought of losing her. That, in my eyes anyway, is true love.

24 JUNE 2015

Last week I found a book on my Kindle that I didn't recognise. I had never even heard of it before and was pretty sure I hadn't purchased it. I meant to email Amazon to tell them there had been some sort of error, but I never got around to it. Tonight I was browsing the photos and videos on my phone and came across a video I had taken of Bea a few weeks ago. She was purring away rolling around with her favourite catnip toy. As I watched, I suddenly realised that during her herb-induced high she had inadvertently been pawing at my Kindle, on which she had been sitting. With three light strokes of the paw she had purchased the mysterious book in question. Thank goodness I hadn't sent that email demanding a refund. Turns out catnip is more educational than I ever realised.

25 JUNE 2015

Mrs Nowakowski had an appointment today with her two-year-old cross breed terrier, Prince. Prince was castrated by us two months ago. He came back in last week unable to pass urine – a medical emergency. Prince had X-rays taken in which contrast material was instilled into his bladder to help visualise his anatomy. On the X-rays, we could see straight away that he had bladder stones, as well as several stones close to the exit point of his penis, the likely cause of his urinating issue. Very unexpectedly, however, the X-rays also revealed parts of the female genital tract – namely a womb. What on earth?

As word spread about this case, a gaggle of vets gathered in front of the X-ray monitor all scratching our heads and looking slightly bemused. Prince was a hermaphrodite! As for people with this condition, it meant he had been born with both male and female sex organs.

He went into theatre later that day to remove the stones and was sent home later in the week. Today he came back in for his recheck appointment and Mrs Nowakowski had decided to bring her whole family with her. It became clear very soon after Prince came into the room that despite our best efforts to explain his condition to Mrs Nowakowski, due to her limited grasp of the English language, she still had absolutely no idea what was wrong with him. Her family unfortunately were also non-English speakers. This was going to be a challenge.

'So, remember when Prince came in and we thought he was a boy and we castrated him?'

After some hand gesticulating and pointing to Prince's penis, Mrs Nowakowski nodded. So far so good.

'Well, then he couldn't pee. And we found those stones in his bladder?'

Another nod, but slightly more apprehensive this time.

'OK, well when we took X-rays we found that he also had a womb. Do you understand the word womb? Uterus?'

A lot of head shaking now, and some raised eyebrows from the accompanying family members.

'Prince has some female organs. It's very unusual but it happens from time to time. He is a girl and a boy,' I offered. Nope, completely lost her now. I paused for a moment, wondering how to proceed. How could I summarise in pigeon English: 'He may need further surgery in the future to assess any communication between his uterus and his bladder, and probably to remove his uterus. Ideally, he needs referral to a specialist surgeon.'

I attempted a lame diagram, but this definitely did not help. I stood back and surveyed my handy work; it resembled a Picasso painting gone wrong and would have been at home in the Tate Modern. I crumpled it up and threw it in the bin.

'He's a lady dog,' I flummoxed them.

'Lady boy?' she repeated.

Eureka.

'Yes, lady boy!' I exclaimed.

There was a sudden loud discussion between all family members in what I assumed to be Polish and a great deal of Prince cuddling.

Mrs Nowakowski turned back to me with tears in her eyes. 'I love him anyway,' she said.

Well, this was a good start. Goodness knows how I would discuss all the other details of his case with her, but at least no matter what happened, Prince(ss) had love on his/her side and you can't really ask for more in life than that.

26 JUNE 2015

Me: What is Boss here for today?

Owner: Oh, he's just having some difficulty with his back legs. I think he's getting a bit stiff.

Me: [Examines Boss, the hyper, bouncy and affectionate Staffie.] Yes, I think he's lost some muscle around his back end and his hips have reduced mobility. We should think about trialling him on some painkillers and tailoring his exercise regime. [Proceeds with discussion about arthritis management with owner, during which time Boss covers me in slobbery kisses as I massage his back and cuddle him.]

Owner: Thanks, that's great. Just before I go, I also wanted to mention that he's covered in ringworm.* My daughter has it too, see. [Owner points to several round lesions on her child's face and multiple small hairless round lesions over Boss's back where I had been massaging him for the last ten minutes.] It's been confirmed by the GP so I just thought I should mention it. The doctor said not to touch him without gloves in case we catch it. It's highly contagious to people, you know.

Me: [Takes some speedy skin samples from Boss then ushers owner out the door and proceeds with immediate decontamination process.]

*Ringworm is a harmless but very contagious fungal skin infection that is commonly shared through direct contact with the skin lesions between children and pets (not to mention the poor parents and members of the veterinary community who spend time with them).

Why do owners always feel the need to mention these things as a parting gift? Would it be too soon to make a dash to Boots for some Canesten Combi?

29 JUNE 2015

Today we put to sleep a dog who had been with us at the hospital for a couple of weeks. Amber, an eight-year-old Staffie, whom we had seen previously for skin issues, was brought in by the police who had visited a man's home when his friends and neighbours reported him missing. He hadn't been seen for six weeks. When the police arrived they found the man had passed away several weeks ago. He had been in the flat with his two dogs when he died and one of them had subsequently died of starvation. Amber was still alive, but barely. The three of them were curled up together on the kitchen floor. Amber was collapsed when she arrived and we fought fiercely to save her. Once she had recovered from the dehydration and was eating small frequent meals, we thought she really had a chance. But she continued to vomit regularly and her demeanour was very dull. We did scans which came back clear, took blood samples which also gave us no answers. We overburdened her with cuddles and TLC. But still she didn't rally. We found no definitive reason for her poor response to treatment and eventually we accepted that she was not doing well and was unlikely to be rehomed in this condition. We told ourselves she had some kind of sinister disease that we were just unable to locate, but the truth was she was dying of a broken heart.

Everyone around the hospital is now very solemn and tearful and the atmosphere is subdued. This tends to happen when one of our rehomers or animals we have fought hard for doesn't make it. Hushed voices, closed doors, red-rimmed eyes. We recover as a community, and we carry on as before, fighting tirelessly for the animals, but each time it happens it leaves a little dent in our spirits.

As usual, my comfort tonight came from Bea, who presented me with a dead bird and two alive but maimed mice when I walked through the door. She always knows when I need cheering up. I spent the following hour cleaning bird poo off my bedding and sofa and chasing mice around my flat. I considered calling crazy-but-lovely neighbour to give her a quick recap lesson on catching them, but thought better of it when I realised how much damage my savage cat had done to them. It's amazing how fast three-legged bleeding mice with half an eyeball can still move. I decided to monitor them overnight and take them to work with me in the morning if they weren't doing well. A vet's job is never done. Still, on the plus side, at least by then I was far too fatigued to dwell on Amber any longer.

1 JULY 2015

Went to visit my nephew at his school today to talk to a class of four- and five-year-olds about being a vet. Super cute. I started the session by introducing them to Digby, the wolf-sized soft toy dog I had brought with me. I'd borrowed him last minute from the X-ray suite at work. Digby earns his keep at PWH by providing trainee veterinary nurses with radiography positioning practice.

The children all seemed keen and warmed to me straight away. Phew. They were busy giving Digby cuddles while I asked who had pets and whether they had ever taken them to see a vet. Lots of raised hands and age-appropriate stories commenced. 'I have a cat called Patch. She had a sore paw'. 'My dog Sam likes to run around and chew up my toys', etc. My nephew then piped up to diligently recount the tale of when 'Auntie Charlotte drove our dead cat home from the vets in the front of her car and then helped us to bury him.' Tough crowd after that.

2 JULY 2015

It was 3 a.m. and the phone rang loudly in my ear. For a moment I thought I was at the airport on my way to a holiday in the Caribbean and the phone was my flight being called. But then I realised I was dreaming. I was instead lying in the vets' flat where I'd dragged myself a couple of hours earlier to get some sleep. I wiped the dribble off my face and tried to sound coherent.

'Hello?'

'Charlotte, it's Sophie. I've got a cat here you need to take a look at. He's not breathing well at all.'

'I'll be right over,' I muttered.

I threw my scrubs on over the top of my pyjamas and stumbled to the hospital. As soon as I got to the emergency room I could see that we were dealing with a very sick cat indeed. He was a Siamese called Mr Bojangles, two years old and extremely skinny. His breathing was dramatically laboured and his mucous membranes blue-tinged. He was panting intermittently, which is always a terrible sign in a cat. I examined him and suspected he had fluid on his chest.

'Get him upstairs into an oxygen cage straight away while I speak to the owner,' I said to Sophie.

I was still trying to switch my brain back on as I went into the clinic to call Mr Pattison through. He was a small bald man with a kind face and timid manner. His facial expression was pained and he looked drawn and exhausted.

'Mr Pattison, Mr Bojangles is extremely poorly. I am very worried about his breathing. Can you tell me a little about his condition? How long has he been breathing like this?'

'He's been unwell the last week or so, picky with his food, you know. I thought it was just because my wife was away in Spain and they are so bonded. But the last two days he's just been lying there, and he vomited this morning. I thought he might die but I didn't know what to do. A neighbour gave me your number and I thought I couldn't leave him any longer.' Mr Pattison started to cry and I handed him a tissue as I patted his arm.

'We'll do everything we can to help him. You've done the right thing bringing him in,' I said.

So often I see animals whose owners have left it way too late to have sought veterinary treatment. I should have seen Mr Bojangles days ago in an ideal world, not now when his lips were blue and he had barely any oxygen left in his body. But it's so complex trying to also contend with an owner's fears and anxieties, and there is a time and a place for chastising people for delaying treatment. This was definitely not the moment for it.

'Please fix him. My wife is autistic, so is our son. They won't cope without him. She has a special bond with him, he follows her everywhere. Please do something!' Mr Pattison was sounding desperate.

I explained that we would try our best to stabilise Mr Bojangles, but the truth was there was every chance he could deteriorate and die in the hospital. I called Mrs Pattison at her husband's request, despite the early hour of the morning. She sounded immediately hysterical, sobbing down the phone.

'Please, please. He's my baby. He can't die without me there. Whatever you do just make him last until tomorrow so I can get back. If I'm there with him he would fight, I know he would. Please, I can't bear it. I've been sitting in the hotel lobby crying for the last three hours. I don't know what to do with myself. Please save him, doctor. Please . . .'

I tried my best to soothe her but I couldn't utter the words she wanted to hear – that he would be absolutely fine and not to worry. I didn't believe this to be true and would be doing her a grave disservice if I lied. I did, however, manage to persuade her to go back to her room and try to get some rest and I told her that I would contact her and her husband as soon as I had any news.

I went up to cat kennels as soon as Mr Pattison had left. Mr Bojangles' breathing had improved very slightly in the oxygen kennel. I took some X-rays which confirmed there was fluid surrounding his lungs. Sadly, the majority of cats with this condition either have cancer or heart failure. His long-term prognosis was looking grim despite his young age. I removed some fluid from his chest and as it came out I suddenly felt more hopeful. It looked like pus. I checked under the microscope and sure enough it was filled with bacteria. Mr Bojangles had an infection in his chest called a pyothorax. This still meant he was an extremely sick boy, but it gave me hope that he could recover. I placed a drain into his chest and sucked out as much of the pus as I could. His breathing had improved considerably now that all that infection wasn't compressing his lungs. I felt an incredible relief mixed with the familiar adrenaline high. I was certainly awake now. The pus would refill and he would need to have his chest drained and flushed daily, but with some strong antibiotics on his side and some intensive nursing care he could get through this.

Once he was stabilised I called Mr Pattison with an update and then went back over to the vets' flat and lay on the bed, sweating in my pyjamas and scrubs and with the heating going full blast. It struck me that central heating in July was not good either for me or for the environment, but I didn't have the energy to move one muscle. I knew I had to get up to sort the inpatients in half an hour and do rounds with the vet on the morning shift.

'Come on, Mr Bojangles, you have youth on your side. You can get through this!' I thought, and then I allowed my tired mind to slip seamlessly from the sick animals in the UK to the blue skies of the Caribbean . . .

4 JULY 2015

It's been three days now since Mr Bojangles was brought to the hospital. I've been arriving early and leaving late for my shifts each day and have probably become overly invested in his case, but I feel haunted by his owners' desperate pleas for help at three in the morning. He's actually doing very well so far. His cheeky character is starting to shine through, despite his unpleasant condition and the painful indwelling chest catheter. I've been assessing his chest fluid each day and he is definitely responding to the treatment so far. What I still don't know is what caused his infection in the first place. Mr Pattison has been calling the hospital every day asking many questions about why and how this could have happened to their young and previously healthy, happy cat. He is not able to afford referral to a specialist and, as with many of our clients' pets, Mr Bojangles is not insured.

Pet insurance is a bit of a gamble, like any form of insurance. You could spend hundreds, if not thousands, of pounds on it throughout your pet's lifetime and if they are generally healthy you may never use it. But if a time comes where you do need specialist care for your furry friend and you can't afford it, the pain and frustration can be immense. Even us vets have to pay vet bills; there are rarely any 'freebies' in this profession, I'm afraid to say. So personally I have chosen to get pet insurance for Bea as if the worst-case scenario happened and I wanted to take her for a second opinion, I wouldn't want finances to hinder that decision.

Without expensive and advanced forms of chest imaging (namely CT and MRI), I could only hope that there wasn't a piece of foreign material hiding in Mr Bojangles' chest somewhere causing the infection. One of the many difficult aspects of this job is not being able to give owners definitive answers. So much of science is based on a combination of evidence and probability. But despite all the advancements in modern medicine there are still many shades of grey, and we simply can't always predict the outcome of a case. So I would continue to treat Mr Bojangles with every available procedure and drug I felt was appropriate, but I couldn't know for sure that at the end of all of it he would be OK. I guess that's where hope comes into it.

6 JULY 2015

Received an understandably hysterical call from James last night during my on-call shift. Bea had found a mouse nest in the garden and managed to bring eight – yes *eight* – mice in one by one through the cat flap. James was now running around our relatively compact one-bedroom flat desperately trying to catch them all. He, like me, has difficulties killing or harming any small creatures, even spiders and flies, and is usually the man for the moment when a mouse wanders into the house. But every man has his limits. I could hear the clatter of Tupperware, the scraping of furniture and the scutter of little feet (I assumed Bea's unless they were giant mice) in among the swear words. I didn't know what to say other than try to soothe James, but I don't think he was really listening.

I had to return to work and the rest of the shift was too busy to call him back. For the first time in my life I was feeling pleased at the thought of getting a few hours' sleep (if I was lucky) in our manky vet flat attached to the hospital, rather than being at home in my own bed with my husband, cat and eight mice.

I arrived home the next morning and all was quiet and calm. No husband, no mice, just a very contented, smug-looking cat. Needless to say, the cat flap had been locked and Bea had been punished for her ASBO behaviour by sending her to bed with no Dreamies. Pets, who'd have 'em?

7 JULY 2015

Sarah left PWH today. I had known for some time it was coming – she had handed her notice in two months earlier and was off to pastures new. I think I had been in denial though. Our last shift together marked the end of an era. We'd worked together most days from my early period of post-graduation terror, when every decision was filled with uncertainty, to our current days of feeling relatively competent and passing our hard-earned pearls of wisdom on to other new graduates. We grew together from tiny tadpoles to medium-sized fish in our big, initially intimidating and regularly chaotic pond. We were by one another's sides through many difficult surgeries, impossibly long afternoons of tedious consulting, traumatic euthanasias and frantic on-call shifts, not to mention through personal traumas and joys, both of which had culminated in copious drunken nights at the pub over the years. It's funny how working alongside someone under sometimes stressful and often challenging conditions can bond you deeply and make you feel like you have known them all your life.

The animal hospital we work in is diverse and filled with receptionists, vets, nurses, ambulance drivers, lab technicians animal care assistants (ACAs) and volunteers from all walks of life. Mostly, we all get along. We are lucky. But there is the odd gem whom you just gravitate towards and they become a friend both inside and outside of the workplace and Sarah was one of those for me. I knew after a rubbish day I could go and have a moan to her and she would just 'get it'. Vets tend to need that, but we don't always find it. It's amazing what a difference friendship makes to your mental health when you work in a job like this. Before she left, Sarah gave me a magnet for my locker which read:

Friends: much cheaper than a psychiatrist.

So true. She will be missed.

8 JULY 2015

My colleague Dan called me this afternoon in a bewildered state. Dan is one of our five designated ambulance drivers who attend the homes of our housebound clients, fetch the animals, and bring them to the hospital for their veterinary appointments. He had returned three black cats to three separate owners following various procedures in the hospital earlier in the day. He had carefully labelled each black cat, both with neck collars stating their name and address, and a label on each basket so there was no risk of confusing them. He returned the first two cats without any problems. When he returned Oscar, the third cat, Mrs Smith (a lovely Caribbean lady who has been a client for many years) became terribly upset.

'That's not my Oscar!' she exclaimed. Mrs Smith was adamant that we had brought her the wrong cat.

I checked the records of what procedure each cat had had in the hospital. Unfortunately, they had all been castrated so we couldn't use this information to tell them apart. They were all similar ages with no identifiable markings. Bugger. If Oscar wasn't Oscar, this potentially meant that we had mixed up all three of the cats. This was a very serious error. How on earth had it happened?! How would we explain this to the other two owners? And how would we tell the cats apart?! It did strike me as odd that neither of the other owners had noticed that their cat wasn't actually their cat, but perhaps they hadn't looked very closely when they arrived home. After several minutes of mild panic, and wondering what on earth to do about the situation, Dan called back again.

'Don't worry, it's all fine,' he said. 'Mrs Smith just forgot to put her glasses on. Turns out it's Oscar after all.'

I could hear Mrs Smith in the background exclaiming, 'Oscar! Oh Oscar, Mummy missed you!'

Thank the Lord. Crisis averted, unexpectedly, by Specsavers.

9 JULY 2015

Summer is a busy time for charity vets, with the RSPCA reporting up to a 50% increase in calls at this time of year. In addition to the plethora of abandoned animals, I've just seen the eighth cat this week to have fallen out of a window. Keep your windows closed, people! Despite the common myth, cats really do only have one life. And a fragile pelvis that will snap into bits like a crunched polo given half the chance.

10 JULY 2015

I discharged Mr Bojangles today. Woohoo! His owners both came to collect him and Mrs Pattison was overjoyed. She really does have a special bond with him. He climbed up her chest and nestled himself into her when she arrived, then began to talk to her in that deep expressive voice unique to Siamese cats. In the eight days since he first arrived I had grown very fond of him and I knew I would miss seeing him sitting by the computer in our cat kennels when we allowed him out to stretch his legs.

'Thank you so much. I will never forget the night I spent abroad thinking that he wouldn't make it and the kindness you have shown us. We are so grateful for everything you've done for him,' she said as she massaged his head and he purred in delight. She produced a laminated photograph of herself with Mr Bojangles sitting on her shoulder like a parrot. I was touched.

'Don't be silly, it's what we are here for,' I replied.

These cases are the most rewarding for me. Young animals who have come back from the brink of death and survived despite the odds. Owners who are filled with love for their pet and gratitude for the help you have given them. They make the bad days tolerable and soften the blow of sadness when cases don't turn out how you'd hoped. They keep me going on the days when I want to give up and think I can't cope with any more sleepless nights or tragedy. They somehow make it all worthwhile.

17 JULY 2015

Been off work for the last few days revising for my certificate exams. All the dreadful memories of years of summer revision, sitting inside reading notes and making revision cards while seemingly the rest of the world was outside enjoying the sunshine have come flooding back to me. If I fail, I won't be struck off the veterinary register or fired from my job but I will feel the shame and disappointment of it just as readily as I would have if I'd failed my university finals, or my A Levels before that. Damn that type A personality. I also can't afford to fail seeing as each exam costs a fortune to sit, not to mention the extortionate fees over recent years for being enrolled on the course in the first place. Unbelievably, the next-door neighbour's twin ten-year-old girls have chosen this very week to practise for their grade five piano exams and the piano is located on the other side of the wall to my desk. You have to love city living. Up the scale, down the scale. Up the scale, down the scale. Combined with the lawnmower and the incessant pigeon cooing, I would definitely prefer to be at work.

Even the beautiful set of new stationery I treated myself to, complete with highlighters in every colour, isn't cheering me up. Are the extra letters after my name really worth all this stress, I ask myself. There is only one way to deal with this situation short of spending the whole day on Facebook, and that's to clean the flat from top to bottom. After a glass of wine, perhaps.

25 JULY 2015

Just returned from a lovely week in the south of France with my husband and his family. A well-earned post-exam treat. While we were there we played a considerable amount of Trivial Pursuit. Coming from a family that is not particularly entertained by board games, I found it amusing and slightly terrifying to witness the level of seriousness with which James's family played this game. It also highlighted my apparent lack of general knowledge. I have clearly spent far too many years learning about dogs' anatomy and cats' physiology to pay much attention to which team won the FA Cup in 1983, or what the capital of Mongolia is. I tried my best to blend into the background and hope that the overwhelming noise of crickets would mask my mute lack of participation, but the most alarming moments always came when the animal or medical questions arose. This would finally be my moment to let my brain full of useless animal facts shine in all its glory. Surely I would know the answers! Surely not.

'How many silkworms does it take to make one kimono?'

'Which colourful crustacean can use its clubbed front legs to strike prey with the force of a .22-calibre bullet?'

Erm . . . pass? (For those of you who care, the answers are 2,000 and a Mantis shrimp or stomatopod, respectively.) Why is it that people always think that if you are a vet you must know every single fact about every single living organism? Crustaceans and insects are definitely not in my remit, unless the insect infects a mammal with some sort of deadly disease, then I would be in with a chance. My brother-in-law had been lumbered with me on his team and the look of disappointment in his eyes still burns brightly in my mind. Turns out my animal knowledge is as limited to cats and dogs as my general knowledge. Sorry 'Team B'. Better luck next time?

27 JULY 2015

Me: What's up with little Spud today?
Owner: He has a lump on his tummy. I'm worried it's cancer.
Me: [Examines Spud.] Oh no, that's actually just a nipple.
Owner: Are you sure?
Me: Positive. He has ten of them, see? [Points to other nipples.]
Owner: Oh. That's a relief. OK, bye then. [Walks out.]

28 JULY 2015

Treated two stray ginger three-week-old kittens today with flea anaemia. Normally fleas are just an occasional nuisance to dogs and cats, but left to multiply without treatment they can cause significant anaemia (deficiency of red blood cells) and even death, especially in sick, very young or old pets. Sadly, one of the kittens arrived collapsed and didn't make it. Diego, my hero, acted as a blood donor for the other one. I really do love that cat, what an absolute star he is. It's one of the most amazing things imaginable watching a ghostly white lacklustre 400g kitten covered in fleas spring back to life as the blood runs into them through a cannula. Their little noses go from white to pink and they suddenly have energy and start wolfing down their food and jumping around like normal kittens should.

We see flea anaemia frequently in this job and it is always frustrating. To have a flea burden significant enough to cause anaemia, there must be hundreds if not thousands of fleas feasting on a kitten's or adult cat's blood, and worryingly this means many more in the animal's home. The fleas drain so much blood that the poor animal is eventually no longer able to function normally. What a dismal thought. In the western world where pets are valued by many as family members, kittens should not be dying from skin parasites that we can easily prevent. Even if we do have Diego the supercat waiting in the wings to save their lives. No biggy. The kitten is off to a foster home next week, all being well, where he will be cared for and weaned and then rehomed once he's big enough. I've called him Diego Junior, obviously.

30 JULY 2015

Received a WhatsApp message from a friend this morning containing three photographs of liquid brown diarrhoea and two of some phlegmy vomit with a bit of grass in it. I quickly ascertained from her message that they were canine faeces and vomit and not her own. Phew. This is not an unfamiliar scenario – owners tend to take endless photographs of their pet's excrement and vomit to show me. It can certainly sometimes be of clinical value, but most of the time just saying 'he has liquid brown diarrhoea' will suffice. I wrote back giving my thoughts on her dog's bad belly, then completely forgot about it until this evening when James asked to look at the photos on my phone we had taken on holiday. My WhatsApp is set to save photos people send to my iPhone camera roll automatically . . . he went right off his spaghetti bolognaise after that.

31 JULY 2015

Me: Gosh, Blossom has gained a good few kilos since we last weighed her, she's becoming quite a curvaceous girl. We mentioned putting her on a diet during your last appointment, how are you getting on with that?

Mrs Gardner: Yes, she likes her food like her mama. [Pats her large belly and then cuddles Blossom, the obese Cavalier King Charles Spaniel, to her ample bosom.] I'm trying but I'm finding it hard, to be honest, dear.

Me: We need to keep an eye on her weight as it could be very bad for her health as she gets older and it makes her arthritis pain worse. What are you feeding her at the moment?

Mrs Gardner: Oh, just the usual. A tin of Pedigree Chum. Twice a day. Plus her dry biscuits, they're good for her teeth. I just pop some in her bowl every now and then throughout the day. She likes to graze, you know how it is.

Me: OK, anything else?

Mrs Gardner: No, not really.

Me: Nothing at all? No treats?

Mrs Gardner: Well, since my Ted passed away, we do like to share my toast and tea for breakfast. And the last vet said I should give her some dental sticks for her teeth. So she has a couple of those each day.

Me: OK. They can be quite high in calories so we are going to need to cut out some of these extras and cut down her portion sizes. Anything else?

Mrs Gardner: Well, she is partial to a bit of cake with me of an afternoon. And every Sunday we have our roast. And she gets a pig's ear from the butcher. Sometimes she likes a bit of fried chicken if she's off the dry biscuits.

Me: Right . . . Is that it?

Mrs Gardner: Yes, dear. Apart from the cheese I give her arthritis tablets in each day. She wouldn't take them otherwise. And we do like to share a rich tea biscuit from time to time if we aren't having cake. We enjoy sharing our food. She looks at me with those big eyes, and I don't like to starve her. That wouldn't be kind.*

Me: [Weeps inwardly.]

---

*In 2018, a study on 'The Future of Pet Ownership' by More Than (Britain's second biggest pet insurance provider) found that obesity, behavioural issues and the rise of designer breeds are all linked to a growing trend of anthropomorphism. Pets are playing an increasingly important part in people's lives, but our humanisation of them is leading to poor nutritional choices and overindulgence. As a nation, we are literally killing our pets with kindness.

3 AUGUST 2015

Saw a fourteen-year-old Pug called Yoda and his owner Mrs Sharpe first thing this morning for a check-up on his breathing. He has chronic bronchitis, an ongoing inflammatory condition which causes a cough and breathlessness. He was doing well over-all and I sent him off with more of his usual medication and told the owner to revisit again in three months' time.

Just after lunch one of the nurses came to let me know that Mrs Sharpe was back at the hospital and that Yoda had been found dead lying in the sunshine in her garden an hour ago. It's 30 degrees Celsius in London today. I rushed down to the clinic where Mrs Sharpe was sobbing over poor Yoda's body. I examined him. His body temperature over an hour after he had died was still 39.9 degrees Celsius; the norm for a dog is 38.3–39.2. I could find no wounds or evidence of trauma. His breathing and general exami-nation had been unremarkable in the morning. Very sadly, it appeared that he had died of heat stroke. I comforted Mrs Sharpe and answered all her questions as best I could but I could see by the anguished expression on her face that she was riddled with guilt. I too felt a sense of responsibility. I had mentioned the heat during our consultation this morning, as I always do at this time of year, but I should have laboured the point.

On my way home, trapped on a sweaty tube carriage that must have been close to 40 degrees, I felt terribly sad for Yoda and the uncomfortable death he must have endured. His facial anatomy had been his enemy today, even more so than on an average day, in addition to his age and chest condition. With several reports in the news this week about dogs dying after being left in hot cars, Yoda served as a stark reminder that we must protect our pets against the heat. With their thick fur coats and inability to sweat, they simply cannot cope. They need shade and a cool fan, plenty of cold water, and to be kept well away from the scorching pave-ments which will burn their little pads. I had to hold myself back from stopping each person I saw on the streets this evening with a panting, hot-looking pooch and telling them to take their dog home and feed it ice cubes immediately. Londoners can be a grumpy bunch, but never more so than when they are hot and bothered. They definitely would not have appreciated the interference, however well-intentioned.

RIP, Yoda.

4 AUGUST 2015

Nearly two months after Ms Armstrong's complaint about the euthanasia of her cat Phoenix, the situation has finally settled down. Ms Armstrong has visited the practice several times for meetings with us. My boss has written three letters back and forth to her and I have also written to apologise for any frustration or lack of communication she had experienced on my part. The Veterinary Defence Society (VDS), an insurance company run by experienced veterinary surgeons on behalf of the veterinary profession who handle many of the claims made against vets, commented recently that the majority of issues that arise in veterinary practices have poor communication at their heart. I can certainly believe that, particularly during emotionally charged consultations such as euthanasias. I have accepted, and so it seems has Ms Armstrong, that we will never view the events or discussions prior to Phoenix's death in the same way. It has served as a reminder to me that however clearly I try to express myself as a vet, and however gentle I feel my approach has been, another human being will not always share the same experience. A client may be listening to me, but not actually hearing or understanding me. And equally, they may be silent when indeed they have strong feelings regarding the matter being discussed.

So should I avoid discussions about quality of life and euthanasia to protect myself from future discord, even if I believe an animal to be suffering? Surely that would go against my code of ethics, and the day that happens will be the day I hang up my scrubs for good. As long as I am a vet, I must always follow my moral compass, whatever the ramifications. Today, though, I can't help but feel a little defeated. After many sleepless nights and long chats with colleagues about this case, I know I need to put it behind me and move on. But there is both a weariness and wariness about my interactions with clients now that wasn't present previously and I'm struggling to shake it.

5 AUGUST 2015

I was working the late shift yesterday. This shift can be very variable which is the nature of the beast. Sometimes there is time for a cup of tea and to help answer a couple of reception calls between emergencies. Other times I find myself still on shift two hours beyond the end of it, writing up cases, calling owners, or finishing up in theatre. Yesterday was the latter. I was making up some medication in dispensary and was in quite a good mood as the sun was shining – a rarity in London. Despite the run of brachycephalics I had seen during the course of the afternoon with heat stroke – luckily none as bad as poor Yoda – all the clients I had met thus far had been friendly and cheerful. Plus I was working with Sally and Frieda again, my two lovely nurse pals, which always improves an average shift. I looked down the end of the corridor and saw Bonnie, the two-year-old Weimaraner who had been spayed earlier that morning, walking out of the lift ready to be discharged. Her owner was waiting in reception. Bonnie seemed a little slow and stumbled as she walked the first few steps. I had checked her half an hour earlier and she had been fine. Suddenly and unexpectedly, she collapsed. I ran down the corridor and immediately started to check her colour, her pulses and her surgical wound. She was pale with a bounding pulse and was bleeding from the wound. A quick abdominal ultrasound scan confirmed blood in her abdomen. A post-surgical bleed. Oh no.

The equivalent of a bitch spay in human medicine is an ovariohysterectomy which requires years of post-graduate training on the surgeon's behalf and a minimum of a three-month recovery period for the patient. In the vet world, we graduate and perform bitch spays from day one. But considering the fact that it is major abdominal surgery, the frequency of post-operative haemorrhage is, in my experience, remarkably low. It is rare for this to happen (and far more common to see disease or complications related to dogs being unneutered later in life), but it is nonetheless what every vet dreads when they do a bitch spay, no matter how many years qualified we are. The vet who had operated on her had gone home for the day, and I was pleased in some ways as it's always much harder to re-operate on an animal you have operated on first time around. You are filled with a sense of dread when you were the primary surgeon that can cloud your ability to focus on the repair. I have been both the initial surgeon when things have gone wrong, and the surgeon who re-operates. The majority of vets with a decent number of years of experience in general practice have encountered post-surgical bleeds, whatever the initial surgery was, although it is still daunting every time it comes along.

After starting Bonnie on a shock dose of fluids and giving her more pain relief, I spoke to the owner and explained the situation. She was understandably worried but I promised to call her as soon as I had any news. I then rushed up to theatre where Sally and Frieda were prepping her for surgery. Less than ten minutes later I was opening Bonnie under anaesthetic and immediately the sea of red hit me. I couldn't see anything and tried not to panic. I took a deep breath and started to suction the blood out and had the nurses on standby to filter it into a special bag for autotransfusion.* It seemed like I had been suctioning

---

*Autotransfusion is a method of providing a blood transfusion to a dog using their own blood, which they have lost through haemorrhage. It is only suitable for certain patients where the blood is considered 'clean' (i.e. not contaminated by cancer or infection in the abdomen) but can be life-saving in certain situations such as this one, especially where there is no option of giving a blood transfusion from another source.

for a very long time before I was able to visualise Bonnie's organs and I started to pack her with as many swabs as I could to stem the bleeding. I couldn't help having a flashback to Zia all those years ago and how helpless and fearful I had felt when I was operating on her. I had surgical experience on my side now and had dealt with dozens of cases of bleeding into the abdomen since that fateful night on-call, but it still haunted me. I managed to locate the source of the bleed and placed a clamp on to the vessel to prevent further blood loss. I followed this with two secure sutures, which I tied so tightly I left indents in my fingers after each knot I placed. After counting out my swabs and check-ing for the tenth time that there was no more bleeding, I closed her up and helped Frieda carry her back down to dog kennels on the trolley. Both Sally and Frieda had stayed an hour beyond the end of their own shifts to help me and I couldn't have been more grateful to them. Lola was on the night-shift duty and when I saw her I gave her a big hug. I felt so reassured just having her there. It's funny how after all these years, the physical presence of another vet you know and trust after a stressful shift can still bring immediate relief. I handed the case over to her. I knew it would be one of those patients I would worry about all night and find myself at work earlier than I needed to be to check on her the next morning.

Sure enough, after a sleepless night I was up at the crack of dawn and on the tube on my way back to work. On the plus side it meant I had avoided the crush of the rush-hour commute as I had travelled in so early. It did, however, feel like I had never left the hospital. I wish I was better able to detach myself from these sorts of cases, but then perhaps if that day ever came, it would mean that I had stopped caring. And if I stopped caring, what sort of vet would that make me? I walked into dog kennels and Bonnie was sitting up happily munching on some breakfast. Thank goodness. After examining her and reassuring myself that everything was as it should be, I called the owner to tell her the good news. Bonnie was going to be absolutely fine.

7 AUGUST 2015

Received a call from crazy-but-lovely neighbour tonight who proudly explained that she had witnessed her cat chasing and catching a mouse in the garden earlier, but that she had managed to stay calm in the face of adversity and had resisted the temptation to call me to come and help. No family members were harmed, they had all stayed on the bench and waited and watched until the cat had run away with his prize. I couldn't face suggesting that next time she try to save the little mouse from his feline clutches. Small steps.

15 AUGUST 2015

Esther appeared in my consulting room today with a rather guilty look on her face. Sophie, my clinic nurse for the day, hovered behind her also looking rather sheepish. It was a busy Saturday morning with lots of emergencies lined up waiting to see me and a hospital packed full of inpatients.

'Um . . . have you heard about the flu cats?' Esther asked tentatively.

'No . . . which flu cats?'

'The RSPCA has seized thirteen cats from an elderly lady's house, all in a terrible state. They have cat flu and are arriving at the hospital any minute.'

Super. And right on cue, there they all were. Thirteen black cats, varying from a few weeks old to several years old, all covered in snot and gunk. The worst affected were unable to open their eyes. They had severe conjunctivitis and ulcerated corneas.[*] If ever there was an advert for getting your pet vaccinated against infectious diseases then this was it.

---

[*]The cornea is the delicate clear outer layer of the eye, less than a millimetre thick. Infection or trauma can cause it to become damaged, which vets take pretty seriously as it always carries the risk of rupturing the eye.

Sophie and I donned aprons and gloves and worked our way through them, weighing them, checking hearts and tummies and mouths and temperatures. We attempted to name them all, mainly after nurses or vets we worked with, and when we ran out of colleagues' names we used the names of some of their children. The last to be examined was a chunky young adult male cat who, having run out of colleagues' children's names by this point, I called Worzel. For those of you who didn't enjoy eighties British television as much as I did, *Worzel Gummidge* is a walking, talking scarecrow character from a children's show. When you name animals on a regular basis, the selection becomes increasingly random, and 'Worzel' just somehow seemed to suit him.

Worzel had severe irreparable ulceration of his left eye and I was pretty sure we wouldn't be able to salvage it. He purred happily when we tickled his chin and he surveyed the scene around him with the pride and contentment of a tomcat who had fathered many of his sisters' and mother's children. Several of the younger kittens were feral and poorly socialised and I suspected they had pneumonia in addition to their phlegm-strewn faces and red-rimmed eyes. Some were feverish. Some emaciated. All were covered in fleas. We piled them into warm cosy kennels in our isolation unit, treated them for parasites, plied them with toys and soft bedding, food and water, and started them all on flu medication. I had high hopes, despite their dishevelled appearance, that at least the strongest ones would make it.

18 AUGUST 2015

I passed my certificate exams! Hurray! I officially have nineteen letters after my name now, which is two more than James. Not that it's a competition or anything. It is a slight anticlimax seeing as it doesn't particularly change my working life in terms of shift length or pay. But after all the hours I have spent writing essays and revising in recent months, I do feel proud to finally have a certificate to practise advanced veterinary medicine. Plus it has pacified my desire to keep learning. Temporarily at least . . .

20 AUGUST 2015

It's been five days now since the cats arrived at the hospital. I have spent more time up in the isolation ward than ever before and definitely more time with them this week than I have with James. So far we have lost four of them, the weakest tiniest ones. The slightly older female kittens looked quite depressed this morning, much to my dismay. The nurses have been amazing, working around the clock to clean them, cuddle them, feed them, give them eye drops every few hours and syringe antibiotic liquid into their mouths. With such intensive work, it's impossible not to become attached to them. One of the tiny ones (aptly named Tiny Tim) is surprisingly still alive and was playing with his ball when I went to see him this afternoon. Worzel was sat in the corner in his relaxed way, contentedly resting with his paws tucked down under his chin in that adorable way cats do. He didn't seem particularly fazed by the fact that his left eye had ruptured and was oozing yellowy-green material. I'm not a religious person, but I said a little prayer to the universe as I surveyed the scene. What a rubbish start to life. I just hoped it wouldn't all be in vain. Come on, little ones, you can do it.

26 AUGUST 2015

Today is National Dog Day! It was set up in 2004 by pet lifestyle expert Colleen Paige to bring attention to canine welfare and encourage people to adopt from shelters. Now it's celebrated annually by all those who care for and about our canine friends.

Today in clinic I saw a total of sixteen wonderful dogs, each one unique and special in its own way. A glorious mixture of big, small, fat, thin, old, young, shaggy, slobbery, long-legged, short-bodied, long-nosed, floppy-eared, black, white, tan and golden, I loved them all! Even the ones who tried to bite my face.

They are our sensitive, loving, courageous pals who just want to love and be loved. Thanks for enriching our lives and being so fabulous, pooches.

#NationalDogDay

(And don't worry, cat lovers, there's an International Cat Day on 8 August, not to mention World Cat Day on 17 February . . .)

27 AUGUST 2015

Update on the black cat flu family. We have four survivors in total. Trying to think positively. Four out of thirteen is better than none. I had to put Tiny Tim to sleep last night after several gloomy days of depression, culminating in breathing complications from his pneumonia. Absolutely gutted. I had grown very fond of the little chap and really thought he might pull through. One of the eight-week-old female kittens made it, although she looks bewildered and lonely without her brothers and sisters. One of the adult females and her 'teenage' (eight-month-old) daughter also survived. They will go off to a rehoming centre together to find their forever home after they have been spayed. They are timid little things and extremely bonded to one another. They should hopefully go on to live long and happy lives together given the chance.

In 2014, the RSPCA released research suggesting that more than 70% of cats in rehoming centres were black or black and white. Black cats notoriously take longer to rehome than cats of any other colour, possibly due to the historic association with witchcraft and the age-old belief that if a black cat walks past it's a symbol of bad luck. Far more disconcertingly in the modern age, there are reports of black cats being rejected by owners because darker-coloured cats photograph badly and don't look good in selfies. When I first heard this I felt a deep sense of despair wash over me. Cats Protection have responded to this problem by creating a Black Cat Awareness day which takes place on 27 October every year to encourage people to rehome them. Black cats certainly have just as much love to give as any other cat. On the plus side, our little black flu kittens are young and thankfully they still have each other. I just have to cross my fingers and toes that they find their forever home quickly.

Then last, but certainly not least, we have Worzel. I knew that amazing beast of a boy wouldn't let me down. He has the potential to be fluey all his life, but he will not let it defeat him. Joyfully one of the senior vets, Jane, operated to remove his eye today and has decided to adopt him. I am over the moon. A happy ending among all the sadness. And a major life lesson: never call a family of ill cats after all the people you work with (or, even worse, their children), only to inform your team one by one that they have all died.

28 AUGUST 2015

Received a text today from crazy-but-lovely neighbour. It read: *I needed you today! Baby bird fell out of its nest in front of me, dead. What do I do with it? I feel bad just throwing it away. It's currently in a pot in my shed.*

After five years of veterinary training and seven years in charity practice I finally feel I am qualified to deal with such questions. I texted back a similar reply to the one I had given previously about the frog and the dead duck: *Leave it to nature.*

31 AUGUST 2015

I arrived for my on-call shift this morning and checked the day list. Winnie was first on the list. I swallowed and felt my pulse rise as I saw the reason: euthanasia. I knew she'd been struggling more and more and that the time was close. But I hadn't realised that today would be the day. Esther is an experienced dog owner. She knows what she's doing and there is simply no way she would let Winnie continue in pain if she felt the bad days were outnumbering the good. Sadly, that time had finally arrived. Despite some weight loss and an increase in her painkiller dose in June, there hadn't been much improvement since I had last seen her. Most dogs her size would be knocked over sideways and need to sleep for a week with the amount of opioid she often had in her system. But it barely touched the sides anymore and lately she had been having episodes of collapse and not wanting to get up in the mornings. She still wasn't making it out of the house for walks very often and was now completely lame on her right back leg. Esther didn't want to put her through any more stints in the hospital, and I admired her for that. They had both had enough.

There is no doubt about it, our pets change us irrevocably and for the better. They give limitless amounts of love to us and in the majority of cases we give it back to them in a symbiotic union. After a short while we cannot imagine our lives without them. They teach us unconditional love and acceptance. They make us laugh and soothe us during life's bleaker moments. Winnie had certainly lived her best years with Esther, and what had come before had ceased to matter. But now the end had come, and all Esther could do was be grateful for every moment they had shared together. We are blessed and privileged to live our lives alongside our furry friends. In the words of one of my heroes and her name-sake, Winnie the Pooh, how lucky we are 'to have something that makes saying goodbye so hard'. After a while, I suppose we all eventually become memories, but our pets live on within us far beyond the end of their beating hearts.

Reception came to let me know that Esther and Winnie had arrived. I could see Esther through the window of the consulting-room door. She was on the floor with Winnie and they were cuddling. She was smiling, stroking Winnie's face, talking calmly to her. Winnie looked peaceful. I was amazed by Esther's strength in the face of the brutal loss she was about to endure. I knew that despite the smile on her face, her heart was breaking. I drew up a syringe full of pentobarbitone, my hand slightly shaking. I prepared the clippers and catheter ready to place in Winnie's leg, as I had done with hundreds of dogs before. I located my stethoscope and placed it around my neck. I picked up a leaflet for Esther about cremation options and pet bereavement, even though I knew she had read them many times over. My movements were measured and steady. The world suddenly seemed to be moving in slow motion. I felt tears prick in the back of my eyes and I shook my head and wiped them away. This was not my moment. I took a deep breath and prepared myself to do the job I had been trained to do. And then I picked up the syringe and walked through the door.

Epilogue

THE HERE AND NOW

Shortly after Winnie died, I stopped writing diary entries. It had been an intense year and the euthanasia complaint followed by Sarah leaving and then Winnie being put to sleep had left me feeling bruised and rather empty. I continued to work to the best of my abilities. Being a vet isn't a job you can do to a 'lesser degree'. You are either there, living in the moment, breathing it in and immersing yourself in it, or you are absent. There is no halfway house. But I could tell that I was starting to feel slightly run down by the sheer vastness of it all. So when, in 2016, I found out that I was pregnant, I felt ready for a new challenge. A break from the animals and the clients and my lovely colleagues. Something different that didn't involve the daily tube commute or the exhaustion of relentlessly hiding my own emotions for the sake of others. I left with my head held high, walking into a new unknown. I had no idea what was in store for me. I will never forget the feeling of walking out of the building I had spent almost every day in for the best part of a decade, not knowing when I would return again.

But in 2017, after nearly a year off work, I did return. There was no doubt about it, going back after having a child was challenging. As a vet you spend years of your life, decades even, dedicating yourself to this one thing. It defines you. When strangers find out you are a vet you are immediately asked a multitude of questions about the job and whether you know what is wrong with their dog's sore paw. It's a topic of conversation among your non-vet friends at parties. It's what stops you attending parties when you are on-call, or too shattered to speak. It's the reason why many vets have long-term relationships with other vets, vet nurses or medics because no one else quite understands the pressures and all-consuming nature of the job. But then suddenly – bang. You have a child and there is something else more important and more consuming and more reliant on you than any puppy or kitten you have cared for. And it's naked, no fur in sight, and you're expected to try and feed this little life-snatcher and do back-to-back night shifts as well as the usual day shifts while recovering simultaneously from the brutality of birth. Shit. Quite literally. Shit all over you, all over your husband, sticky mustard seeds up the baby's back and down her legs and in her hair, and in your hair, while the poor cat sulks in the corner as all the commotion is most certainly disturbing her usual sleeping routine. And the screaming! I knew I was blessed to have this bundle of juicy new-born perfection in my arms, but there is a reason why the SAS use sleep deprivation and audio recordings of babies screaming as a form of torture. For months after the birth I wondered how on earth I could do this mother thing. How could anybody do it? It's surely an impossible task meant only for super heroes. It was only those magical glassy-eyed looks of love during three a.m. night feeds where it felt like we were the only people still awake in the world, and the incomparable feelings of immense love for her, that kept me going. Well – that, coffee, friends and wine.

I learned a great deal of new skills when I was on maternity leave, although I did find myself drawing on my veterinary skills on an almost daily basis. It's amazing how wrestling with an angry Jack Russell prepares you for changing a nappy one-handed while pinning a wriggling baby down with the other. I was already an expert at drinking half a cup of tea and leaving the rest to go cold, so that felt like business as usual. And my cast-iron stomach, built up over years of being exposed to noxious substances, helped me not to vomit when my baby was sick in my mouth. It was reminiscent of the time I was in theatre and a pyometra exploded in my face. For the record, it's a close call but I would say that having vomit in your mouth is just slightly preferable to having pus in your mouth.

Gradually, bit by bit, I began to surface for air. I started getting more sleep and remembering that I did have a life before this tiny wriggling dictator came along and took over. And that former life involved animals, and using my brain, and being a vet. When my daughter was five months old, I did an online course on feline endocrinology in an attempt to get back into the swing of things. It was one of those interactive ones where you log in and they ask questions during the session and you submit your replies. My daughter fell asleep ten minutes before it. Fab. I even had time to make a cup of tea. I sat down with my laptop ready to go. Time to use some of those brain cells again! Wishful thinking. A few minutes after it started, the familiar cry of hunger/teething/generally being a nocturnal creature filled the room and the remainder of the session was done with babe in arms.

When I sent a summary of the important things I had learned to my boss to pass to the rest of the team later in the week, I missed out the highlights of breastfeeding and screaming-baby-bouncing while learning about the new treatments available for thyroid disease. How I longed for the pre-baby professional development course experience. A soggy sandwich and peaceful snooze at the back of a dark lecture theatre sounded like utter bliss at that moment.

By the time I went back to work when my daughter was ten months old, I felt I had achieved some sort of equilibrium between life and being a mum. I had managed to get a vague handle on this motherhood malarkey and had come to terms with the constant feelings of inadequacy and guilt. I had even begun to really enjoy my time 'off' and I had met a whole new group of incredible and supportive women – my 'mum pals' – without whom I would surely have fallen into a sleepless baby-vomit-induced coma months before. It was the first time in my life for a very long time that my group of friends did not include vets. And then it dawned on me. I knew how to be a vet and I had learned how to be a mother. But how on earth was I going to be both? I had not operated in nearly a year. I had only held a handful of consultations on my keeping-in-touch days and felt woefully out of practice. What happened if I got to work to do the job I was so familiar with twelve months earlier, and I couldn't do it?

I spent the evenings in the run-up to my return feverishly reading through old university and certificate notes and watching YouTube videos of surgeries I had done a hundred times over. I do sometimes feel like women get the raw end of the deal. Leaving your career is hard, especially when you've trained for years to get to where you are. But coming back after having a baby is even harder. I was wracked with a sense of guilt. Guilt about going back and leaving her. Guilt about becoming a part-timer and having to leave work on time, even though, as it transpired, this still never happened. Guilt about always feeling frazzled and not having enough time for Bea, for my family, for my patients, for my clients and colleagues, let alone for myself.

After a large number of tears – both mine and my daughter's – I dragged myself out of the door and on to the tube, shook myself out of my baby coma, and walked back through the door of PWH.

The team was slightly different, though still as hard-working as ever. Several of my colleagues had moved on to pastures new during my absence, leaving a hole behind them that was difficult to fill. With increasing numbers of animals to treat, the pressure to help as many pets as possible using limited charity resources had never felt so urgent. Before long, I found myself right back in the middle of the drama and chaos of it, and I had to admit I had missed it.

My first day in theatre I had a cruciate surgery. No easing me in gently with a cat castration, or a wound to stitch up. Thankfully, Lola was on standby to offer moral support and we scrubbed in together. On my second day in theatre I had two ferret spays, a rabbit spay, a pyometra and a cat that had eaten her owner's hair extensions, which were now lodged in her gut. By the end of the day I felt like I had never left. Over time, leaving my daughter got easier and being back at work helped me to revive a part of myself that had been dormant for a year. It may not always sound like it, but I love my job, and my break away had confirmed that.

As with many professions, there were parts of the job I had been dreading returning to. Euthanasias are never pleasant but, for me, the hardest part of being a vet has always been the euthanasia refusals. This seems to be more of an issue in the charity sector where clients don't feel any financial pressure to make a euthanasia decision. The cat that has had an aortic thromboembolism (like a stroke) and is paralysed, dragging its back legs and yowling in terrified agony with no chance of recovery. The dog with a bone tumour with a hopeless prognosis who is in too much pain to take another step forwards. The cat that suffered pelvic trauma and is now completely incontinent, so sits day after day in the hospital having his bladder manually expressed, waiting for the owner to make that decision. The dog with end-stage arthritis who reeks of ammonia from the urine dribbling around his back end, who is on the highest dose of pain medication and can no longer get to his food bowl unless his owner carries him to it. Being a vet isn't a licence to kill. But it's certainly a licence to help end suffering.

Then there are the best bits. During my time away on maternity leave, it was the first time in over a decade that I hadn't had daily exposure to treating animals. I missed the cuddles and handling them, talking to them and just hanging out with them. I missed the cute puppies and kittens, but way more than that I missed the angry snarly elderly toothless dogs and cats with one eye, three legs and matted fur. I hadn't anticipated having an actual physical yearning to be around all those crazy creatures. And it was more than just the animals. I missed my colleagues. The banter, the case discussion, the catch-ups while stitching up a wound, the giggles and the academia. I missed the complex medical cases and the buzz I would get when I successfully treated an animal and they came back to see me in full health. I missed the clients and their sometimes hilarious, sometimes insane, often heartbreaking stories. I missed the chit-chat. I missed the sad lady who came in each week carrying her Chihuahua in one arm and pushing her disconcerningly realistic looking fake baby in a pram with the other. I missed the lovely gentleman in a wheelchair who lost his legs to diabetes, but would do anything to help treat and control his dog's diabetes. I missed the eccentric lady who was convinced that her dog had tiny spiders crawling all over him, no matter how many times we had explained to her that they were fleas. I missed the client who insisted on dyeing her Maltese Terrier's hair bright pink every month because it looks 'cute', even though the poor little pooch has allergic skin disease. I missed the two sisters that came in with their scruffy terrier Ted, who spent the entire consultation finishing one another's sentences in between bickering about how often he had vomited, whether he had eaten his breakfast that morning, and how many times he had done a poo that day. I missed Mr Johnson with his elderly cats, repeating their names after every sentence, and Ms Cruz with her stories about spiders and honey-roasted ham. I even missed the clients' shopping lists of all the ailments they wanted me to treat in a ten-minute consultation period.

When I met my publisher in the early stages of writing this book, I travelled into central London and walked through a part of town where men and women wear suits and there are stilettos and brogues galore. I wandered along in my flat sandals and jeans and felt utterly out of place among this sea of well-clad city professionals. It reminded me that working in an office and wearing anything other than scrubs would be a completely alien concept to me. The vet world is unrefined and every day brings something different. It is unglamorous to the max. At any given moment I may have bodily secretions belonging to an animal in my hair, down my trousers or even in my eye. I once spent a whole afternoon in theatre wearing underwear that had been drenched in cat urine through my scrubs. I didn't have a spare pair of knickers, nor would I have had the time to change into them even if I had. You become fairly desensitised after a while. But walking around the city seeing how other people go about their daily work life reminded me that I wouldn't have it any other way. I can't picture myself working in an office and, despite the inconvenience and unpredictability of veterinary hours, I would take my cat-urine soaked underwear over a pair of stilettos any day. There is never a day where I can predict what will come through the door next, and there is always a surprise lurking around the corner. Every time I think I have 'seen it all', I am proved wrong. I have no idea whether I will stay in the charity sector or indeed continue my working life in the insanity of central London. I often dream about the relative calm of life in the countryside and wonder whether life there might provide more balance. But wherever my path takes me in the future, I realise now that the vets I met on my travels all those years ago were right. Being a vet is a privilege. Despite the stress, anxiety, salary stagnation and long hours, it is still the best job in the world. Or at least the only job I can imag-ine spending the rest of my life doing.

RESOURCES

FOR POTENTIAL OWNERS
WISHING TO ADOPT A PET:

Contact your local veterinary surgeon for advice including information about local Kennel-Club-registered pet sellers.

Check animal charity websites or call them for breed and suitability information. You will also find information on general cat and dog care on these websites.

Battersea Dogs and Cats home – Visit battersea.org.uk

Blue Cross – Visit bluecross.org.uk/rehome-pet or call **0300 790 9903**

Cats Protection – Visit https://www.cats.org.uk/adopt-a-cat or call **03000121212**

Celia Hammond Animal Trust – Visit celiahammond.org

Dogs Trust – Visit dogstrust.org.uk or call **0207 837 0006**

New Hope Animal Rescue – Visit newhopeanimalrescue.co.uk/blogs, find them on Facebook or Twitter (@MailNewHope) or emal newhopeanimalrescue@hotmail.co.uk

PDSA – free puppy information pack and puppy contract. Visit pdsa.org.uk/taking-care-of-your-pet/looking-after-your-pet/puppies-dogs/getting-a-puppy or call **0800 917 2509**

RSPCA – Visit rspca.org.uk/findapet

Contact your nearest animal rehoming facility and arrange a visit, or browse the animals available on their websites.

FOR THE LATEST REPORTS ON THE
PUPPY SMUGGLING SCANDAL:

Visit www.dogstrust.org.uk/news-events/issues-campaigns/puppy-smuggling/ or call **0207 837 0006**

FOR INFORMATION ON BREED SPECIFIC LEGISLATION (BSL):

Blue Cross petition to end BSL
bluecross.org.uk/our-campaign-end-breed-specific-legislation

RSPCA campaign and information on BSL
www.rspca.org.uk/getinvolved/campaign/dogownership/bsl

The SaveABulls campaign – veterinary-led information on BSL
thesaveabulls.com

FOR VETERINARY STUDENTS OR VETS IN NEED OF MENTAL HEALTH SUPPORT:

The Samaritans is available 24 hours a day and calls are completely confidential. Email jo@samaritans.org or call **116 123**

Vetlife operate phonelines 24 hours a day for vets at crisis point or in need of emotional support. Call **0303 040 2551** or visit vetlife.org.uk/mental-health/

Vets4vets are a confidential support group for vets in the USA. Call **(530) 794-8094** or email vets4vets@vinfoundation.org

HOPELineUK offer support, practical advice and information to young people considering suicide and advice if you are concerned about someone you know. Call **0800 068 41 41**

CALM aims to prevent male suicide in the UK and offers confidential help. Call **0800 58 58 58** (every day between 5 p.m. and 12 a.m.).

Royal College of Psychiatrists leaflet on 'Feeling Overwhelmed' vetlife.org.uk/wp-content/uploads/2015/10/Feeling-over-whelmed.pdf

ACKNOWLEDGEMENTS

Writing this book would not have been possible without the support of many people in my life.

First, I would like to thank my work family, past and present, for making me into the vet I am today. To Caroline for her friendship and support over the years. To Cristina and Katy who have battled through it all with me since the beginning. To Candice for helping me to overcome my fear of the scalpel, Alison T for guiding me through many a sticky situation, and all the other vets who have been on this crazy rollercoaster with me. To all the wonderful nurses I have worked with over the years – if I named them all the list would go on for several pages. We couldn't do the work we do without you. To the receptionists, ACAs, lab technicians, animal welfare officers, van drivers and all the other staff members who have kept me sane. Thank you. I truly believe I stumbled upon a special bunch of people when I started my job as a charity vet. The work that continues to be done 24/7 by every staff member on the 'shop-floor' at the hospital is quite frankly awe-inspiring. Wherever I work in the future I will never forget the years I have spent working, laughing and crying alongside you all.

Thank you to Winnie and Diego (and their owners) for letting me tell their stories. Winnie is gone but never forgotten.

Thank you to my university buddies for getting me through the relentlessness of vet school and helping me not to quit on multiple occasions. To Kate W and Kate J in particular, whose friendships have endured the test of time and geography. You both know how much you mean to me. And to my childhood friend Kate M for encouraging me to speak to the vets we met on our travels all those years ago.

Special thanks to James, Alison, Kate W, Caroline and Will for reading through early edits of this book and making sure I wasn't writing anything too crazy.

Thank you to Jojo for putting me in touch with my literary agent, Cathryn Summerhayes. And to Cathryn for pursuing the idea of this book and encouraging me to go for it. Thank you to Charlotte Hardman and Fiona Rose at Hodder who saw potential in me and have been extremely supportive throughout the process of writing this book.

And, most importantly, thank you to my family. To my wonderful family-in-law who have always been so kind. Nick and Iliana, I will find you the perfect pet one day! Michael and Moira, you are my second parents and have supported me through every triumph and hurdle of my veterinary career thus far. To my siblings, Will and Emily, who are always there for me and have motivated me to keep going through the highs and lows of writing this book. To my parents Sarah and Lyle who made all of this possible and have been by my side cheering me on since the day I was born. Life as working parents of three children can't have been easy, not to mention caring for the endless stream of pets we insisted on adopting. And thank you to my entire family for listening and not feigning complete boredom while I brainstormed different ideas and book title options. Special thanks to Moira for helping me finally to settle on the title *Animal Matters*.

Thank you to Snowy for being the best pet a child could ask for, and for teaching me how to care for another living creature. And to my daughters Molly and Mabel whose reliable daytime naps allowed me the opportunity to research and write this book. And last but not least, thank you to James, my partner in crime, who gave me the courage to embrace this project and put up with months of me being constantly distracted and half-absent as I feverishly scribbled down my thoughts and memories. I quite simply couldn't have done it without you.